From Psychiatric Patient to Citizen

From Psychiatric Patient to Citizen

Overcoming Discrimination and Social Exclusion

Liz Sayce

First published in Great Britain 2000 by
MACMILLAN PRESS LTD
Houndmills, Basingstoke, Hampshire RG21 6XS and London
Companies and representatives throughout the world

A catalogue record for this book is available from the British Library.

ISBN 0–333–69889–4 hardcover
ISBN 0–333–69890–8 paperback

First published in the United States of America 2000 by
ST. MARTIN'S PRESS, INC.,
Scholarly and Reference Division,
175 Fifth Avenue, New York, N.Y. 10010

ISBN 0–312–22733–7

Library of Congress Cataloging-in-Publication Data
Sayce, Liz.
From psychiatric patient to citizen : overcoming discrimination
and social exclusion / Liz Sayce.
p.   cm.
Includes bibliographical references and index.
ISBN 0–312–22733–7
1. Mental illness—Public opinion.   2. Discrimination against the
mentally ill.   3. Stigma (Social psychology)   4. Mental health laws.
I. Title.
RC455.2.P85S29   1999
362.2'0422—dc21
99–16944
CIP

This book is printed on paper suitable for recycling and made from fully managed and
sustained forest sources.

10   9   8   7   6   5   4   3   2   1
09   08   07   06   05   04   03   02   01   00

Printed in Hong Kong

Contents

List of Abbreviations

AA	Alcoholics Anonymous
ACAS	Advisory, Conciliation and Arbitration Service (UK)
ADA	Americans with Disabilities Act 1990
APA	American Psychiatric Association
ASA	Advertising Standards Authority (UK)
DBTAC	Disability and Business Technical Assistance Center (US)
DDA	Disability Discrimination Act 1995 (UK)
DfEE	Department for Education and Employment (UK)
DoJ	Department of Justice (US)
DREDF	Disability Rights Education and Defense Fund (US)
DSM	Diagnostic and Statistical Manual (US)
DSS	Department of Social Security (UK)
EAP	Employee Assistance Program (US)
ECT	Electro-convulsive therapy
EEOC	Equal Employment Opportunity Commission (US)
FBI	Federal Bureau of Investigation (US)
HEA	Health Education Authority (UK)
HUD	Housing and Urban Development Department (US)
INS	Immigration and Naturalization Service (US)
JAN	Job Accommodation Network (US)
MRI	Magnetic Resonance Imaging
NAMI	National Alliance for the Mentally Ill (US)
NARPA	National Association of Rights Protection and Advocacy (US)
NHS	National Health Service (UK)
Nimby	Not in My Back Yard
NSF	National Schizophrenia Fellowship (UK)
SAMHSA	Substance Abuse and Mental Health Services Administration (US)
SSI	Supplemental Security Income
SANE	Schizophrenia: A National Emergency (UK)
WHO	World Health Organization

Acknowledgements

I would like to thank all the user/survivors of mental health services, in the US and UK, who have generously shared their thoughts with me, and to acknowledge everyone who has spoken openly, in any context, about their experiences of distress, depression or madness. Without people prepared to be open, often at considerable risk, there would be no movement for challenging discrimination on mental health grounds.

I am enormously grateful to all the user/survivor and disability leaders, policy makers, advocates, lawyers, mental health professionals and academics, in the US, the UK and beyond, who have shared their views and time with me and in many cases gone to considerable trouble to assist my research.

Among those who have contributed directly to this work, I would like to mention Len Rubenstein, previously Executive Director of the Bazelon Center for Mental Health Law, who guided me through my Harkness Fellowship research in the US; the Bazelon Center for its tremendous hospitality; Vida Field, Judi Chamberlin, Michael Allen and Len Rubenstein for invaluable advice on different drafts; the Harkness Fellowships for making this work possible; my ex-colleagues at Mind for stimulating and creative debates; my mother, Olive Sayce, for heroic assistance with proofreading; and Jane Elliott for kindly translating a Chinese disability discrimination law to satisfy my curiosity. The views expressed here are, however, mine alone.

This book is partly about how to break down barriers to enable user/survivors to be part of different 'communities'. At best, communities can provide us with many things, including personal identity, a common purpose with others, support, friendship, feedback – and a sense that we belong in a social world. I am part of a generation of women who have built networks of friends, replacing older geographical communities. I would like to thank my family and my 'community'.

The author and publishers wish to thank the following for permission to use copyright material:

Australian National Mental Health Strategy Community Awareness Program, an initiative of the Australian Commonwealth Department of Health and Aged Care for the mental health poster (*The defence didn't stop him. Neither did mental illness*) reproduced in Chapter 11.

Brown Brothers for the Ellis Island illustrations in Chapter 3.

Gary Brookins for his cartoon, depicting a service user as an axeman, first published in the *Richmond Times-Dispatch*, Virginia, May 1997, and reproduced in Chapter 10.

Health Education Authority for the Mind postcards reproduced in Chapter 11.

Every effort has been made to trace all the copyright holders but if any have been inadvertently overlooked the publishers will be pleased to make the necessary arrangements at the first opportunity.

Introduction

I don't want half a life. I want a life (Lionel Aldridge, ex-Green Bay Packers player and mental health user/survivor, 1995).

This book is about creating social inclusion for people diagnosed with a mental health problem. It addresses one central question: how, and on what basis, do we move beyond the physical desegregation of hospital closure programmes towards the chance of full participation in social and economic life?

The primary focus is neither on mental health treatments nor on the organisation of services to deliver them. As the attention of mental health policy makers and planners has moved across complex issues of service organisation – managed care (in the US) and local commissioning (in the UK) – the question of how to have 'a life', rather than a service, has sometimes been eclipsed. This book aims to fill a gap in the debate.

The first part of the book establishes a conceptual basis for challenging social exclusion, by outlining a vision of inclusion (Chapter 1), an alternative 'nightmare' scenario of spiralling exclusion (Chapter 2), an examination of discrimination, including multiple discrimination, as it affects user/survivors (Chapter 3), and an analysis of the potential and pitfalls of four current models for tackling discrimination or 'stigma' – the brain disease model (Chapter 4), the individual growth model (Chapter 5), the libertarian model (Chapter 6) and the disability inclusion model (Chapter 7).

The book's second part examines different avenues for creating change, highlighting the achievements for mental health user/survivors of the world's most advanced disability discrimination law (Chapter 8), the limitations of law (Chapter 9), the significance of public and political debate in framing law and policy (Chapter 10), the potential of educational and media work to influence public attitudes (Chapter 11), and the impact of grassroots work and alliances on making inclusion happen (Chapter 12).

The conclusion suggests strategic ways forward.

1

The book is based on several sources: guided discussions with
user/survivors, lawyers, advocates, policy makers, disability
activists and mental health professionals, in the UK and in 11
American states and the District of Columbia, as well as with individuals working at national level in both countries; knowledge
derived from direct experience working in mental health policy
and campaigning in the UK and, to a lesser extent, the US; and a
study of the literature, especially user/survivor literature, on
discrimination and how to overcome it.

Lessons in history and geography

This book is based primarily on research undertaken in the US and
UK in the late 1990s. It also makes reference to work undertaken in
Europe more broadly and in Australia and New Zealand.

It may be tempting to think that by looking more widely – at
other moments of history, other countries or cultures – we might
find clear solutions for discrimination on mental health grounds
already established.

Warner (1985) has shown that, in 'developing' nations, recovery
rates for people with schizophrenia are generally higher than in
'developed' nations because people do not lose their status, work
or role in their community. In some African countries, people may
participate in rituals that mean they receive attention – unlike the
common European or American practice of depriving people of
their usual company and support (Warner 1985).

Some have argued that certain native American healing ceremonies – like Navajo 'sings', in which someone who is unwell
performs with the extended family and contacts, sometimes for 5
or 9 nights – can effectively restore people experiencing mental
health problems to active life in their community (Bergman,
quoted in Benedek 1995). In Navajo culture, it is said to be
'harder to become isolated, to feel that there is no one looking out
for you' (Benedek 1995).

In the Saami community in Lapland, helping someone through
the experience of psychosis is seen as important for the whole
community and not just the individual (Nergard 1997).

Developed market economies may have much to learn from
developing nations, but we cannot necessarily import Navajo
'sings' or Nigerian village norms unchanged into the South Side of
Chicago or London's Hampstead. We should also beware of ideal-

ising other times, other places. If pre-asylum England supposedly had its village idiots happily accepted in the community, it also espoused Christian notions of madness linked to possession and sin (Dain 1992). In some present-day African countries, such as Zimbabwe, madness is widely believed to derive from witchcraft or 'ngozi', that is, punishment for wrongdoing by ancestral spirits, and those affected are feared and devalued (Ndlovu 1997). To return to native American peoples, they have been mixed in their treatment of people deemed 'mad'. The following example relates to a Pahvant Chief in late 19th-century Utah:

> The greatest tragedies of [Chief] Kanosh's life came from his family. He had four wives, three of whom died tragic deaths. Julia, his first wife, became insane while young, and the tribesmen, according to custom, tied her to a wild horse and dragged her to death during the absence of the chief (Daughters of Utah Pioneers 1994).

A complex set of material and cultural conditions is likely to be significant in determining how a people defines its 'mad' and how accommodating it is towards them: for instance, whether and how it defines 'perfection' of mind and body and their opposites, on what basis it distributes resources and what other cultural preoccupations it links to 'madness'. Oliver (1990) notes that practices in relation to physically disabled people vary enormously between cultures – from infanticide to endowing disabled people with special spiritual gifts. He argues that the level of 'surplus value' in the society, together with the ideology underpinning the redistribution of wealth, may influence how accepting it is to disabled members. Foucault (1967) argues that madness is constructed, and treated, according to the preoccupations of the age. For example, in medieval England, madness was seen in religious terms, as a sign of the end of the world; during the 'great confinement', it was seen through the lens of a condemnation of idleness, as European economic crisis made inactivity appear to be the major threat of the moment. More recently, it has become linked to a preoccupation with crime.

Foucault goes further, suggesting that we have constructed the polarity of reason and madness and, by implication, could deconstruct it. Yet the earliest known assessment tool for identifying 'madness' was produced by Cicero in the 1st century BC (Darton 1998a). Across history and culture, distinctions are drawn on the issues of madness, distress and sanity – albeit differently framed.

'Madness' ranges in meaning from spiritual power to demon possession or sickness, and 'sanity' from reason to emotional or spiritual wholeness, but there is little evidence of societies that hold no distinction at all.

Attempts to dispense with these conceptual divisions almost invite resistance. People have observed and named differences in thought, feeling and behaviour, and will only eradicate one type of distinction by creating another. For instance, re-evaluation co-counselling questions the whole construction of mental illness and mental health, seeing it as a divide that creates a fear of being thought mentally ill – which keeps us all 'in line' (see Ch. 5). There may be many reasons – ethical, political, artistic – why a society would do well to reduce the fear of being thought mad. Yet co-counselling replaces the standard mental health divide with another: people are either stuck in their patterns of distress, which are caused by oppression, or they are able to discharge the distress and move on. Even those most opposed to the gulf between madness and sanity tend to create new distinctions.

We can, of course, soften the sharp edges of these polarities, stress that there is a fine line between madness and sanity, that it is we who have constructed the definitions – so we can construct them differently. We can question the whole basis of current diagnosis (Bentall 1990, Boyle 1993) or set up much more complex models (see Ch. 1). But, however refined the conceptual model, society around us will use it to define many of the people experiencing what we currently call 'serious mental health problems' as different (see Ch. 11). The most pressing task facing the mental health world is to establish that being 'different' does not mean having any lesser value, rather than expecting prejudice to fall away by arguing that difference does not exist.

The study of the historical and cross-cultural variables involved in the treatment of disabled people generally, and people with mental health problems in particular, is incomplete. It is beyond the scope of this book. Further work is needed on how lessons in social inclusion from developing countries can be adapted to market economies and how, within nations, majority cultures can learn from minority communities. Some practical initiatives have been established, for example the use of traditional African puberty ceremonies in Britain, which appear to help young black men with mental health problems to negotiate the path to adulthood (Chief Omalade, personal communication, 1997). But evaluations are few.

Lessons from the American and British experiences described in this book cannot be exported, ready made, to different parts of the world. Such a practice can verge on the absurd as, for example, when traumatised women in a Ugandan refugee camp in the 1990s were offered the help of a Western dance therapist. They rejected her assistance in favour of being given a small plot of land and tools to dig and grow food (Ugandan mental health worker, personal communication, 1997). However, the ideas in this book may be of interest in countries facing similar dilemmas to those seen in the UK and US. 'Nimby' (not in my back yard) campaigns, for instance, are remarkably common:

• in Hong Kong, in 1992, a plan by the Hong Kong Mental Health Association to set up the Amity Day Centre in a neighbourhood community centre met with 'vigorous actions' by local people. Would-be attendees were followed and harassed (Mental Health Association of Hong Kong 1993).

• in New Zealand, a 1997 survey of mental health user, relative and provider organisations found that 84% identified as a problem community 'alarm' about the siting of both community housing and acute in-patient units. Ninety-eight per cent said that stigma generally was an issue for their organisation (Peters 1997).

• in the Tyrol, local politicians led a campaign to stop any mental health services from being opened, arguing that there were no people with mental health problems in their area (population 80,000) (European Day of Disabled Persons 1995).

All countries that have segregated people in long-term institutions, and which have subsequently decided to mix the 'sane' and the 'insane', are subject to 'nimby' opposition. This applies to considerable chunks of the world (Kemp 1993).

Other trends currently affecting numerous countries include the restructuring of welfare (where it is significantly developed) and the growing influence of global corporations, including pharmaceutical companies that have vested interests in promoting particular models of thinking about mental health and mental illness (see Ch. 4).

Britain and the US

The US merits study because it has both the most comprehensive disability discrimination law in the world covering psychiatric disability (see Ch. 8) and some of the most extreme social and economic polarisation (see Ch. 2).

Britain has followed certain American developments (see Ch. 2) but Britain is also European by tradition and therefore more committed to ideas of social welfare and social responsibility. This can bring more paternalistic services than in the US, less choice and fewer individual rights: 'Europeans don't understand rights', as one American law professor put it to me. However, it also brings greater equity. American mental health services include numerous high-quality and innovative employment support, advocacy and other services. Yet during the blizzard of 1996, people residing in St Elizabeth's Psychiatric Hospital, Washington DC, sat in their coats as money could not be found to repair breakdowns in the heating system. In Britain there are far fewer user-run services or services to support individuals to obtain work: Peck and Barker (1997) found that only 22% of London's mental health NHS Trusts had any scheme to support users in getting work and that those focusing on the open employment market were 'universally poor'. However, far fewer British users are entirely without health care or without heating in hospitals (see Ch. 2).

Britain is of interest since it could at best combine the most effective of American human rights traditions and the most inclusive of European notions of collective responsibility. At worst, it might combine European paternalism with American patterns of social exclusion. If it achieves the first, it could create a synthesis of traditions of use to other European countries as they restructure welfare and health care.

Some commentators have argued that discrimination on mental health grounds operates differently in Britain from elsewhere: in particular, 1990s Britain was swept by a 'moral panic' about violence committed by users of mental health services following a number of highly publicised homicides (even though the incidence of homicide had not increased; see Ch. 3). Yet while Muijen (1997) argues that constant media linkage of mental illness and violence occurs only in Britain, and Ramon (1996) that a demonisation campaign has occurred 'in the United States, in Britain, but nowhere else (at least for the time being)', the truth appears more complex.

Violence is firmly linked to mental illness in media coverage in both the US and UK (see Ch. 3), and also in New Zealand where, for example, journalists reported a 1996 mass murder in Tasmania in terms of the probable psychiatric disorder of the perpetrator. The fact, when it emerged, that he had no mental illness did not receive a similar degree of media attention (Mental Health Commission 1997). Different specific 'panics' have emerged in different countries, states and cities, often attaching the fear of madness to other potent concerns of the moment: violence in the workplace – almost none of which in fact is perpetrated by people with mental health problems (see Ch. 8) – an American panic fuelled by one heavily publicised case of a 'crazed' Post Office employee who turned a gun on colleagues; infanticide – a Chicago panic, stemming from the killing of a child by a woman with mental health problems, which exacerbated concerns about the safety of public agencies' decision making; and random street violence, a British panic, fuelled by the emblematic, but highly atypical, British case of Christopher Clunis, a man with mental health problems who killed a total stranger in a London Underground station.

In different localities, 'stories' emerge and succeed each other in varying patterns, not in line with actual trends in crime or other social phenomena but according to subtler cultural shifts. Some countries have a stronger record in including positive 'stories': in Italy, the push for 'democratic psychiatry' enabled users to appear somewhat heroic, of interest for their successes in getting out of institutions rather than for more 'demonic' qualities (Ramon 1996). British and American experiences are not, however, unique, and globalisation of the media is likely to make 'stories' increasingly international, as framed by more influential nations. This could mean a spread of moral panics – rather as movie watchers internationally are influenced by American films, which make frequent links between madness and violence (Wahl 1995).

This book aims to identify anti-discrimination approaches developed in the US and the UK, with a particular emphasis on synthesising individual and social rights and responsibilities. The lessons may be of relevance elsewhere.

Personal starting points

To tackle social exclusion not only means changing our views on who is or is not 'employable', or changing our laws on who has a right to live where. It also means changing our conversations in bars – challenging discrimination at the micro, personal, level of how we think and act.

For myself, I came to think about what discrimination on mental health grounds meant through examining a number of layers of experience.

As a teenager, I found myself suddenly subject to intense attacks of anxiety – I felt that I could not breathe, sometimes that I could not speak. I had no idea what caused or triggered these experiences and was quite unable to explain it when asked. Then I started counting the cornflakes and the lettuce leaves I ate, as my weight dropped beyond the fashionably thin. I believed that the image I saw in the mirror was horribly fat – a somewhat mad view, with a weight of under 6 stone. My own stance was that I was fine, and I fought off lurking fears of going mad with a degree of success most of the time. My partner of the time worried that I was 'having a breakdown', a notion that I brushed aside a little too desperately. The truth was that I was terrified of losing control, of being 'mad', and could only cope by pushing away attempts at help from parents and friends.

Images of madness in our culture make it starkly clear that it is best avoided or denied – not just because the experience can be alarming, but because it is hard to see oneself simultaneously as 'crazy' and as a valid person with a liveable future. As one woman with a dual diagnosis of mental illness and drug problems put it to me:

> It's more OK to be an addict than to be mentally ill. We'd seen the Betty Ford Clinic – but nowhere had I seen the welcome wagon for mental illness. I thought of the poorhouse next door, from my childhood. It was a mental institution. I assumed I'd be institutionalised for life. I was pleased when the mental health service said I couldn't get a service from them because I wasn't clean and sober. I didn't want to deal with what I thought about mental illness (user/survivor, Texas, 1996).

I was lucky. With very supportive family and friends, and the opportunities of education and interesting work, I found a way through my problems without ever taking on the status of psychiatric patient. Denial in that sense worked for me. For many, it does not. Seeking help can bring an excruciatingly complex mixture of advantages and disadvantages: someone, at best, to listen and offer support, but life chances potentially jeopardised permanently by a psychiatric record.

I do not share the experience of compulsory detention or treatment, nor of discrimination on the basis of a psychiatric record, although I want to be an ally to those who do. But I was affected, in my struggle with some strange experiences, by the fear of what it might mean to be 'mentally ill'. Discrimination on mental health grounds affects millions because so many people fear being 'on the wrong side of the line' and go to such pains to make it clear – not least to themselves – that, even when distressed, they are not 'mad'.

It is useful for anyone wishing to increase social inclusion for user/survivors to think through how they identify themselves and why. It eases communication with others whose experience is different and improves the chance of working together effectively. However, it is not straightforward in the context of current choices of concepts and language.

User/survivor organisations often welcome anyone identifying as a 'survivor' , which can be defined very broadly: 'a person with a current or past experience of psychiatric hospital, recipients of ECT, tranquillisers, and other medication, users of counselling and therapy services, survivors of child abuse' (Survivors' Poetry 1996). 'Survivor' is an immensely positive and hope-inspiring word. Yet in most contexts (from earthquakes to cancer), talk of 'survivors' implies the existence or possibility of those who did not survive. In the mental health field, we need language, and a movement, that includes and respects the non-survivors – those who commit suicide or live their whole lives in high-security hospitals. The aim is to assure value for people who are on the so-called 'wrong' side of the line – and not merely to help as many as possible to cross to the 'right' side (see Ch. 7).

'User' or 'consumer' of mental health services is also a constraining concept. At this point of history, post-'community care' and with a new emphasis on disability rights, we are broadening the focus of challenge from power imbalances within mental health services to those in society as a whole. For this, we should consider promoting such terms as 'disabled' or 'socially excluded'. The social model of disability holds that a person is disabled if he or she is, for example, blind, and experiences barriers and exclusion as a result. The term is not limited to those who 'use' blindness services nor to people who are 'surviving'. It covers everyone

affected by discrimination on the grounds of the supposed imperfection of disability. It allows for transforming negative associations into positive ones, through disability pride.

A wide movement, rooted in new language, could be combined
with people identifying themselves much more specifically – 'I am
socially disabled and a survivor of forced treatment' or 'I am
excluded on mental health grounds and a user of forensic psychiatry services.'

My own first brush with the fear of madness did not prepare me
for dealing readily with discrimination on mental health grounds
when it appeared later, in different guises. Through discussions
with colleagues in a variety of mental health organisations, I
found that many of us had at times called in sick, with vague
descriptions of being ill in bed, implying that we were physically
ill when we were in fact distressed. People suggest many reasons
for this concealment: privacy; or the fear of being thought less
genuinely unwell than if you had, for example, tonsillitis; or the
fear of being treated differently in the future. All can be attributed
to discrimination. Take privacy. One might wonder why we want
to keep distress more private than a stomach upset. In either case,
it is possible to limit discussion to the initial statement rather than
go into huge detail about the precise digestive problems or
emotional nuances. Physically ill people, in general, telephone
work without a second thought and say they have food poisoning
or flu. The reason for keeping emotional distress quiet is not a
generalised desire for privacy but a desire for privacy about stigmatised states. At present, that includes a limited number of physical illnesses (such as AIDS) and almost all sorts of emotional and
mental health problem.

Or take the fear of being thought a 'skiver'. The issue at stake in
deciding whether or not to call in sick is not whether the problem
is physical or mental/emotional but how severe and incapacitating
it is. To make a physical/emotional distinction is simple discrimination (Faulkner and Sayce 1997). People who do not define themselves as user/survivors might be better allies for those who do, by
deciding to be more open – not leaving all the culture-changing
responsibility to the user/survivors.

At the same time, as a manager and campaigner in the mental
health field, I encountered some who believed that when someone
was 'stressed' or 'distressed', he or she should automatically be
excused core work activities. This is discrimination of a patronising
form. Employers do not have to accommodate distress where this

seriously impedes productivity (except where subsidies or substitution arrangements are used to encourage work by people unable to work at 100% capacity; see Ch. 8).

A further personal dimension was added when I became involved with a partner who has a diagnosis of manic depression. I do not, however, think that this makes me a 'carer', because this is a mutual relationship, not one in which 'care' goes one way, and not one involving 'burden' (an offensive term that should be dropped from research design and discussion).

Several excellent accounts exist of relatives and friends being allies for user/survivors. For example, Jennings (1994) publicised the ways in which her daughter, who had been abused in childhood, was 'revictimised' in psychiatric hospital. She was never private, never free of the fear of invasive forced treatment, sexually harassed again and not believed when she tried to report abuses. Clara Buckley, whose son Orville Blackwood died in seclusion in Broadmoor Hospital, highlighted in the mass media the plight of black men in British secure hospitals. However, I only know of one study on the contributions that user/survivors make to their relatives and friends. Greenberg et al. (1994) found that where they lived together, 50–80% of relatives/friends said users contributed by doing household chores, shopping, giving emotional support, listening to problems, providing companionship and providing news about family and friends.

The term 'carer' also assumes that one party is more competent. Yet no one teaches most of us how to be effective allies for user/survivors, even if we work in mental health. Friends and relatives can feel far from competent, and need to learn from user/survivors, who are often more 'competent' in responding to distress because of having been through the ravages of thinking and feeling that way themselves (see Ch. 1). Instead, if relatives receive advice from anywhere, it is usually from professionals, which can have a depowering effect on user/survivors.

Getting involved with someone with mental health problems can raise concerns in other people. As one woman put it to me, 'I wasn't his carer, I was his girlfriend. I liked being his girlfriend. Some friends didn't understand that.' I encountered no disapproval, but I was aware of the possibility. Will people think that this relationship reflects some problem of mine, making me 'gravitate' towards someone with a mental health problem? Will the more psychodynamically orientated of them think I am seeking someone to play out my depression for me – or to give me the power of a 'caring' role? Will they seek to assure me that there is a solution – in therapy, or drugs, or whatever – thus implying that life with a mental health problem has to be unendurable? None of this happened, but the images run deep because getting involved with someone diagnosed with mental illness involves breaking a taboo against keeping our distance from 'madness' and those it affects (see Ch. 3). The relatives and partners of user/survivors need discussion and information to support them in noticing discriminatory views in themselves and others, and in rethinking and challenging them.

The literature on 'carers' tends to neglect these issues in favour of a discussion on the need for information and general support. It includes claims that 'carers' need more rights to be involved in decisions about care and treatment, perhaps even to be able to purchase it on a user's behalf. I would find it intrusive to make decisions on someone's treatment unless it was clear that they had wanted this. What if the user/survivor has fallen out with you? What if you are a relative who has exploited them, and from whom they need protection, rather than decisions supposedly in their interests? Far from extending relatives' rights over user/survivors, we should secure relatives' and friends' rights to their own support – and reduce their automatic role in decision making, for example, by abolishing the 'nearest relative' provisions of the British Mental Health Act 1983 in favour of a general provision for advocacy by someone of the user's choosing.

If we want employers, neighbours and the 'general public' to drop discriminatory attitudes towards people diagnosed mentally ill, we have to be able to do so ourselves. Considering that it is statistically probable that virtually everyone will know at least one user/survivor in their lives – whether they know it or not – the question of how to be an ally merits increased attention.

A final layer of my experience was being part of the British Government's Disability Rights Task Force (1997–99) and co-ordinating Mind's 'Respect' campaign; while I wrote this book, I was also taking practical steps to reduce discrimination.

In clinical work, it is generally agreed – although not always practised – that work needs to be rooted in a theoretical and research base. In policy-influencing work, while there are a few handbooks on how to campaign (see, for example, Lattimer 1994, Shaw 1996), many campaigners proceed on the basis that they know 'what is right'. Urvashi Vaid has written a trenchant critique of this approach, which she believes was one of the reasons why the American gay and lesbian lobby had achieved only 'virtual equality' by the mid-1990s. They were, she says (criticising herself alongside others) so concerned with arguing the finer points of the policy 'line' that they failed to analyse and pursue the strategies that would actually effect change (Vaid 1995).

In Britain in the late 1990s, views differed among mental health advocates on the best approach to the first Labour government for nearly 20 years. Some thought the strategy should be to be extremely non-confrontational – based on the argument that the government's concern with news management would mean that they would 'cut off' anyone inclined to embarrass them publicly. Others thought that the best way of influencing a government concerned with news management was through the news, otherwise one could have as much access to government as one liked but no power base from which to negotiate. Literature on these dilemmas exists, suggesting that the second position is more likely to be effective, as long as it is conducted with full communication and respect for government, only speaking publicly about a complaint after making the point privately and giving decision makers ample opportunity to respond. If they do not, or if they go back on a commitment, public comment is usually needed, and it may assist decision makers in their negotiations with other government departments. As Shaw (1996) puts it:

> Silence in the face of a politician's initial betrayal sends a clear message that your constituency feels itself too weak, too confused, or too afraid to merit respect.

He argues that being flattered by being invited to meet mayors or other dignitaries is no substitute for strategizing. It is vital not to confuse access with influence (Vaid 1995).

The idealism that drives campaigns is not always matched by a strong debate on methods. Campaigning, by its very nature, sometimes oversimplifies – the current situation is wrong, a new law would be 'the answer' and so forth. Once one stands back, theorises and examines evidence, it can become more difficult to 'sloganise'; conversely, however, the slogans can become more grounded in what is likely to work best with different target groups. One aim of this book is to provide a chance to stand back.

Choice of language

In mental health, as elsewhere, the US and the UK are divided by a common language. In the US, people who are, or have been, diagnosed with a mental illness tend to define themselves as consumers, survivors or ex-patients. Each term carries a very different implication. Consumers may seek help from mental health services (even if critical of them and/or deeply involved in setting up consumer-run alternatives). Survivors have survived the system, as well as any original problem, and may not choose to 'consume' (or be consumed by) it again. 'Ex-patients' is a more neutral term. The term 'c/s/x' (consumer/survivor/ex-patient) is used to be deliberately inclusive.

In the UK, 'consumer' was rejected as implying more purchasing power than was really available, and the pertinent distinction is between 'users' of services and 'survivors'. In this book, I generally use 'user/survivors' (the British equivalent to c/s/x) or refer to people by the terms they choose. No term is without pitfalls.

The word 'disabled' may have the unfortunate connotation of being 'unable', but it has been reclaimed (see Ch. 7). In the US, many people favour 'people first' language – a 'person with a disability, rather than a 'disabled person' – in order to avoid making the individual totally identified with the impairment. In the UK, disability activists often prefer 'disabled person' on the grounds that to say 'with a disability' suggests that it is a thing, like blindness, whereas 'disabled person' stresses that society is doing the disabling, it is a process. I follow the British choice – except where quoting Americans – although both reflect clearly argued positions. The British have not widely adopted any equivalent to the helpful American notion of 'people with psychiatric disabilities', perhaps because the British mental health movement has come later to cross-disability work. I use 'socially disabled' or 'psychiatrically disabled' to describe people who face exclusion on the grounds of actual or perceived mental health problems.

A thorny question is whether to talk of 'stigma', 'discrimination', 'social exclusion' and/or other terms. Oliver (1990) argues that disabled people, generally, have not found stigma a useful concept because it has been unable 'to throw off the shackles of the individualistic approach to disability with its focus on the discredited and the discreditable'. The legacy of Goffmann's work on stigma (Goffmann 1963), he argues, has been a focus on individual self-perception, and microlevel interpersonal interactions, rather than widespread and patterned exclusion from economic and social life. 'Stigma' has not provided a rallying point for collective strategies to improve access or challenge prejudice. Instead, the disability movement has turned to structural notions of discrimination and oppression.

In relation to mental health, Judi Chamberlin (personal communication, 1997) has argued that the concept of 'stigma' is itself stigmatising, implying that there is something wrong with the person, while '"discrimination" puts the onus where it belongs, on the individuals and groups that are practising it.'

A national strategy to combat discrimination against people with mental illness in New Zealand stated:

> Years of research into public attitudes and stigma have not led to the development of effective models for change... Whereas stigma attaches to the consumer, discrimination results from actions of others. If placed in a human rights framework, there is clear evidence that widespread discrimination is exercised against people with mental illness. More importantly, that framework also offers a well-tested methodology for identifying and resolving discriminatory practices (Mental Health Commission 1997).

The mark of shame, it can reasonably be argued, should reside not with the service user but with those who behave unjustly towards her or him.

The questions raised by these critiques are not merely semantic. Different conceptual models point to different understandings of where responsibility lies for the 'problem' and different prescriptions for action. For example, by using the term 'racism', we focus our attention on the collective and individual perpetrators of discrimination. This construct leads us to solutions based on challenging the power of racist ideas and actions, for example, rendering discriminatory actions illegal, or embarrassing, through the media, those companies that practise institutional racism. If, instead, we construe the problem in terms of the stigma of being black, our attention shifts, to the self-image and perceptions of the black individual. Our solutions may then centre on encouraging black people to have higher self-regard, to shake off their sense of inferiority or insecurity.

This analogy is instructive. Given the dominant discourse of 'racism' to which we are culturally attuned, a solution based primarily on expecting black people to change their self-perceptions comes across as victim blaming. It is reminiscent of the 'he's got a chip on his shoulder' form of analysis, which in liberal circles is likely to be seen as unacceptable. It appears to be a diversion from tackling the material realities of racism: the interconnected disadvantages of high levels of school exclusion, unemployment, low income, a lack of inherited wealth/property, poor housing and ill-health. (For example, in Britain in 1995, unemployment among black African men was 30.8%, among black Caribbean men 23.3% and among white men 9.5% (Bloch 1997); see also Modood *et al.* 1997 for inequalities across education, housing, health and other policy sectors.)

In the field of mental health a number of terms have been coined that are equivalent to 'racism', for example, 'sanism' (Perlin 1995) and 'mentalism' (Chamberlin 1977), both meaning discrimination on mental health grounds. These have not gained general currency. This leaves a conceptual gap, which continues to be filled in part by the long-used concept of 'stigma', but increasingly also by the competing concepts of discrimination and social exclusion (see, for example, Corrigan and Penn 1997, Mind 1997a). While in one sense these may be less potent than 'racism' or 'sexism', as they do not emphasise the highly specific discrimination faced by mental health service users, they do shift the emphasis from the victims of unfair attitudes and treatment to the individual *and collective* perpetrators.

It is important to note that some commentators attach multiple meanings to the term 'stigma' in ways that may lessen the risk of victim blaming, for example, including patterns of social exclusion as part of 'stigma' (Link *et al.* 1997; see also Sayce 1998a). The New York-based National Stigma Clearing House has also used a broad definition of 'stigma' effectively to challenge the unfair depiction of mental illness that runs through the media, film and product marketing (see Ch. 11). Attaching multiple meanings to the term 'stigma' can, however, blur different issues – social, political, economic and individual (Sayce 1998a). There is, in addition, a danger that a word that originally meant a brand of disgrace on an individual, and which has been much used to examine individual adaptation or otherwise to the 'disgrace', will keep pulling our thinking back to the psychological experience of shame, and away from the meanings added by later academics and activists, viz social and economic patterns of exclusion.

An article on stigma by Hayward and Bright (1997) demonstrates these dangers vividly. The authors discuss whether the benefits of being 'labelled' mentally ill outweigh the costs. They argue that the acceptance of illness may be a valid goal of treatment, 'but only if effects on self-image are also addressed'. They go on to ask, 'how can we alleviate the negative effects of a *feeling* of stigmatisation?' (my italics). The problem is, however, not just one of 'feeling': it is one of actual discrimination (see Ch. 3). Helping users to change their 'specific stigmatising (and therefore self-denigrating) beliefs' through cognitive therapy, as Hayward and Bright advocate, is no substitute for reducing the level of discrimination. Users are most likely to shed their sense of shame if we succeed in attaining a society in which they are treated with greater value than at present (Sayce 1998a).

This analysis may be objected to on the grounds that 'discrimination' is also problematic. In particular, it has two meanings that are easily confused: it can be used to mean either unfair treatment, as I have used it here, or treating people differently, that is, being 'discriminating'. The latter is not a negative term; it can indeed be very positive for service users, who do not generally want to be treated 'the same' as everyone else, any more than women want to be treated 'the same' as men or Moslems 'the same' as Christians.

This ambiguity can be averted by a simple definition of the term 'discrimination' to mean unfair treatment. Discrimination is a useful word because it creates resonances with other fields, where it has already been established that discrimination is unethical. The most obvious alternative to 'discrimination' – to develop the use of a more specific term, such as 'sanism' or 'mentalism' – has other drawbacks. In the current climate, new 'ism' words are often seen as demanding of individual rights rather than offering contribution, as self-seeking rather than communitarian, as out-of-date, 'politically correct', 1960s thinking. Even if these ideas are misguided – people challenging sexism, for example, often being more interested in establishing new ethics than in being self-seeking in existing terms – at this moment of history, they render the coining of new words risky. 'Discrimination', and 'social exclusion' are powerful because they enable user/survivors to benefit from a so-called 'common sense' that has already been established: that discrimination is unfair, that everyone should have a chance to contribute and be involved. For potential pitfalls of the term 'social exclusion', see Chapter 2.

CHAPTER 1

A Dream of Inclusion

Is madness interesting?

> I want to be able to talk to someone in a pub and say 'I have been mentally ill' and for them to say 'that's interesting, what did you experience?' (user/survivor, UK, 1997).

More commonly user/survivors report that people change the subject, suddenly find they have to leave or back out of future contact. For example:

> It's worse than having a sexually transmitted disease. If you have gonorrhoea, everyone wants to talk to you about it. If you have a mental illness they want to avoid you (user/survivor, San Antonio, Texas, 1996).

The first person's dream was to close the social distance that 'sane' people so habitually place between themselves and those they see as mad or weird. In this dream, people with mental health problems would automatically be seen as part of the communities in which people operate: the pub, the mothers' group, the health club. And everyone would have learnt – at first reluctantly – that having a mental health problem does not have to stop people from contributing, as friends, colleagues, partners or parents.

In this imagined future, the term 'community care', as meaning 'not located in a hospital', would have fallen into disuse. It would seem laughably euphemistic, given its currency at a time when user/survivors were so massively excluded from 'communities' ranging from the workplace to the family.

A dream of inclusion

If we pursued this dream vigorously, we might in 20 years expect to find that laws and policies to ensure fairness had ushered in serious change. During the late 1990s, 70–90% of Americans and Britons classified as disabled by mental health problems, and of working age, were economically inactive, that is, neither working nor seeking work (Mancuso 1996, Labour Force Survey 1997/8). In the general working-age population, by contrast, 70–90% were economically *active* (Convery 1997). In Britain, only 13% of those with long-term mental health problems were actually working, compared with 35% of disabled people generally (Labour Force Survey 1997/8). For some groups – black users and those with a criminal history – the rate was far lower. Yet evidence is accumulating that people with long-term mental health problems can work effectively, given the right support and 'adjustments' (for example someone to talk to or a quiet space). Anthony *et al.* (1995) found no relationship between psychiatric diagnosis and work skills. Symptoms were, however, more severe in the unemployed: work acts as a protective factor. Moreover, with support on the job, employment rates can be increased significantly for those with severe, long-term difficulties (Matrix Research Institute 1995). Bond *et al.* (1997) found that, in all the experimental studies reviewed, a mean of 58% of clients in supported employment programmes achieved competitive employment, at minimum wage or above, compared with 21% of controls. While not all user/survivors can work full time, and some need considerable support to enable them to work, effective work and achievement are possible, and positively beneficial, for those with long-term mental health problems (Shepherd 1984). On the basis of the evidence to date, one London NHS Trust works from the premise that 'given the correct support and training, employment can be an option for everybody', 'employment' meaning anything from a full-time job to a few hours of paid work a week. (Lewisham and Guys Mental Health Trust Business Plan 1997).

By 2020, the extraordinarily high economic inactivity levels among user/survivors could be slashed – through laws requiring access, backed by workplace policies, management training and advice, and intensive support for people seeking and maintaining work. If we devise effective social security protections for people with fluctuating difficulties, subsidise employers to cover any individuals who cannot work to 100% capacity or who need periods of time off sick, introduce user-run substitution systems so that people can cover for each other when unwell, and ensure that capital is available for user-run businesses, then we could bring the economic inactivity rate down not simply to the average for disabled people but to the level for the population at large. In current terms, that might mean at least 87% of user/survivors working rather than the appalling current figure of 87% out of work.

When deinstitutionalisation began in the 1950s, sceptical voices declared that most patients would be unable to live outside hospital. Forty years later, accumulated evidence showed a range of benefits of community service developments over long-term institutionalisation for most users (Stein and Test 1980, Reynolds and Hoult 1984, Mosher and Burti 1989, Muijen *et al.* 1992, Leff *et al.* 1996). Muijen *et al.* found that no controlled trial showed hospital care to be better on any variable. Leff *et al.* found that, 1 year after patients were discharged from long-term hospital care to community houses, they had more people they regarded as friends and significantly improved community and domestic skills, and they also valued their greater freedom in the community. Only 2 out of 737 ended up in prison. In this context, even those most opposed to hospital closure, like Marjorie Wallace of SANE (Schizophrenia A National Emergency), began to talk of the *minority* for whom 24-hour staffed accommodation was needed (see, for example *Daily Telegraph*, 17 January 1998). The case in favour of employment opportunities for user/survivors – in terms of health benefits, human rights and evidence of practicability – is equally compelling.

While a few 2020 reactionaries would still hold to the view that the 'crazies' should never have been allowed into the workplace, most would be afraid to say so. Many would no longer be convinced of it, having become used to co-working with many disabled people and having found points in common with, for example, colleagues diagnosed with schizophrenia. As with allowing women to be managers or physically disabled people to be college students, there comes a time when resistance seems so outdated that it goes underground, becomes more subtle and ultimately loses some of its potency.

In this constructed future, the work ethic would not be the only force for social inclusion. Other activities – being a parent, an active member of a church or mosque, or a politician – would be as open to user/survivors as would paid employment. It would be commonly understood that while most users might need no 'adjustments' in the environment to enable them to participate, some would: for example, if someone became distracted by hearing voices in a parent–teachers' meeting, she might request a short break to enable her to drown them out by listening to a personal stereo, or to go outside and talk back to them. She would expect this request to be accommodated if possible. The presumption in business and community organisations would be that disabled people belonged in the group – in every group – and that it was everyone's business to know how to talk and work with them. Communicating with someone who was deaf or who had mental health problems would no longer be left to the 'experts'.

This generalised confidence could take the edge off people's fear of madness. Old stereotypes – like the myth that people with mental health problems are in general violent – would gradually lose their grip on the public imagination. Measures to prevent violence in society would be both more sophisticated and more equitable than at present, no longer singling out those with 'mental disorder' for preventive detention but instead taking a range of preventive action with anyone with a propensity to violent crime – the man who beats his wife when he gets drunk, the gang members who fight.

In this changed culture, newspapers would no longer dare to publish insinuations that people with mental illness contribute significantly to violent crime, nor to publish disproportionate numbers of pictures of black user/survivors in connection with violence (Sayce 1995a). The 'big, black and dangerous' stereotype would be a matter for historical study only.

Dreams or flights of fancy?

This scenario appears idealistic, on the grounds, perhaps, that 'people will always have their fears and prejudices against people they see as "other"'. It is, however, worth remembering that 40 years ago many white people in the Southern United States genuinely believed that they could hold on to segregated education and lunch counters. Thirty years ago, most British people did not envisage that disabled children would have begun to be effectively included in mainstream education (Clough and Lindsay 1991). It would be irrational confidently to state now that the segregation of user/survivors – in mass unemployment, poverty, 'sheltered' work, 'sheltered' housing and the like – will always be needed. Equally confident assertions about other groups have led to retractions and apologies. For example, in 1963 Governor Wallace of Alabama physically blocked the door of the University of Alabama to its first black student for the sake of the TV cameras and his re-election prospects. In 1979, Wallace stated to a black church congre-gation, 'I think I can understand something of the pain black people have come to endure. I know I contributed to that pain and I can only ask your forgiveness.' In 1980, he publicly renounced his segregationist views.

It is the contention of this book that we can gradually overcome the tendency to segregate, keep a distance from, people with mental health problems. Obstacles and setbacks will be numerous but need not stall the whole enterprise. There are a number of forces that may support this social change.

The reduction of stigma and discrimination on mental health grounds is becoming an increasingly high policy priority in a number of countries. The Australian Government has undertaken a major public education campaign. The New Zealand Govern-ment introduced an anti-discrimination strategy based on lessons learnt from other marginalised groups who have achieved change, such as people with HIV/AIDS. The American Substance Abuse and Mental Health Services Administration launched leaflets and a Website devoted to the subject (Sayce 1997a). Governments are building partnerships with business, educational institutions and other agencies to spearhead change.

So why is the reduction of discrimination of interest to policy makers?

- Mental ill-health accounts for 28% of the years lived with a disability in all world regions apart from Sub-Saharan Africa. In those countries where lifespan is increasing, and deaths from communicable diseases reducing, the conditions presenting most challenges are those that are long term and disabling. Suicide has become the tenth leading cause of death world wide, approximately level with road traffic accidents. Mental ill-health accounts for 10.5% of something called, rather negatively, the 'total global burden of disease', calculated by combining years of life as a disabled person, years of life lost and mortality rates. Projections suggest this could rise to 15% by 2020 (Jenkins 1997).

- Reports from the World Bank, World Health Organisation (WHO) and Harvard School of Public Health have raised the profile of mental health with the United Nations (UN) during the 1990s. In 1995, Boutros Boutros Ghali, UN Secretary General, stated: 'Priorities must change... To secure mental health for the people of the world must be one of the objectives of the United Nations in its second half century.' In 1996, the UN set up an international awareness initiative, 'Nations for Mental Health'. It was proposed that governments should undertake mental health impact evaluations of all major policy proposals, equivalent to reviews of environmental impact (Jenkins 1997).

• Governments concerned about reducing the incidence of mental ill-health might turn their attention to the social and economic costs of leaving whole sectors of their populations socially excluded. Wilkinson (1996) has shown that, in countries such as the US and UK, where disparities of income and wealth are wide (and widening), social cohesion suffers; they have higher rates of violent crime and morbidity than do more cohesive societies such as Sweden or Japan. He argues that the intervening variable between relative poverty and ill-health is chronic social stress:

To feel depressed, cheated, bitter, desperate, vulnerable, frightened, angry, worried about debts or job or housing insecurity; to feel devalued, useless, hopeless, isolated, anxious and a failure; these feelings can dominate people's whole experience of life, colouring their experience of everything else... [these psychosocial processes] are important not only from the point of view of those low down the social scale who suffer them most, but also because the deterioration of public life, the loss of a sense of community, and particularly the increase in crime and violence, are fundamentally important to the quality of life for everyone.

Many different theoretical models have been proposed to enhance participation and inclusion. Examples are the 'stakeholder' society, in which risk is shared, inequality kept in check and individualism stemmed through active intermediary organisations lying between the individual and the state (Hutton 1997), and communitarianism, emphasising the need for group and individual responsibility in order to balance rights (Sandel 1981, 1996). If political initiatives emerging from any of these ideas prove effective, among the newly 'included' would be people living with mental distresses that arose from the very conditions of exclusion.

• Governments concerned to increase economic activity rates among disabled people – and to reduce the costs of disability benefits – swiftly realise that unemployment tends to be higher among people with mental health problems than any other group of disabled people (Labour Force Survey 1997/8). This suggests the potential to make most impact in this area.

- For people who have already developed mental health problems, social exclusion can cause massive further damage and health care costs. Discrimination continues even after mental health problems have been effectively treated, and is associated with relapse and an intensity of ongoing problems (Link et al. 1997). Many user/survivors fear even applying for jobs because of an – often justified – fear of rejection (Read and Baker 1996, Link et al. 1997). Long-term poverty reduces social networks that could be protective (Bates 1996). If even middle-class Americans are increasingly 'bowling alone' rather than socialising in groups (Putnam 1996), the chance for unemployed people with mental health problems to join many social activities is ruled out by poverty and rejection (see Ch. 3). Physical illness stemming from social exclusion can exacerbate mental distress, as people become trapped in vicious circles from which it is ever harder to escape. Conversely, in societies in which there is a 'social consensus for recovery', and user/survivors are included, serious mental health problems such as schizophrenia are less long lasting (Warner 1996).

- The cost-effectiveness of mental health services is reduced by the prevalence of discrimination. Even the best laid professional care plans can be thwarted if the person's mental health is undermined when his or her parental rights are unfairly terminated or friends cease to call (Link et al. 1997, Sayce 1997a).

- Discrimination puts some people off seeking help at all, not only because some fear admitting to themselves that they may have a 'mental illness', given the loss of status that they (usually correctly) predict will follow, but also because they may previously have encountered aspects of the mental health services that reflect discrimination in the wider society rather than providing a haven from it. For example, a woman may have been admitted to a psychiatric ward and experienced sexual harassment or assault: over 50% of British acute units reported such problems for women in-patients in 1997 (Sainsbury Centre for Mental Health/Mental Health Act Commission 1997). She therefore feels unsafe to return to psychiatric services ; 'I'd feel safer sleeping on a park bench', as one young woman put it (Sayce 1995b).

These fears of services impede key policy goals: to ensure that people with severe mental health problems do not 'slip through the net', to maintain continuity of care and to reduce the number of crises. Escapees from services may rather be subjected to repeated compulsory admissions, which are neither satisfactory for them nor cost-effective.

- Mental health service developments are routinely thwarted by public opposition (see Ch. 3). 'Nimby' campaigns can lead service providers into expensive legal wrangles and delays to projects (Repper et al. 1997).

- Discrimination can weaken family and friendship groups. They pick up the stigma at one remove – having to decide what to say about their friend or relative's 'problem', and sometimes sharing in poverty or social isolation.

A growing movement

However compelling the reasons for dismantling discrimination, it will not happen without pressure.

The user/survivor movement has grown from small beginnings, such as the late-19th-century Alleged Lunatics' Friend Society, to thousands-strong national, regional and global networks (Campbell 1996). Some aims have remained constant: the Alleged Lunatics' Friend Society believed that 'each patient should have a voice in his own confinement and care, and access to legal representation' and wanted to 'convert the public to an enlarged view of Christian duties and sympathies' (cited in Plumb 1994). One member, John Percival, stated that patients were first crushed 'and then discharged to live a milksop existence in society'. User/survivors have reframed their demands, but the substance of complaints is not radically altered, partly because in the intervening 100 years human rights and dignity have still not been fully achieved.

User/survivor activism has, however, brought changes that could hardly have been imagined even 30 years ago. Chamberlin's idea of creating user-run alternatives to mainstream psychiatric services (Chamberlin 1977) has been turned to the reality of user-led drop-ins across the US and beyond; user/survivors have been openly employed as psychiatrists and nurses; their contribution to the quality of clinical work has been recognised by academics and professionals alike (Mowbray *et al.* 1997); and users have been directly involved in policy making, for example through the 1990s' British Government's Mental Health Task Force and Independent Reference Group on mental health. Moreover, more and more people are choosing to 'come out' about their experiences (Faulkner and Sayce 1997). At a 1996 public demonstration in Philadelphia, where users marched openly on the streets for parity between physical and mental health insurance cover, Joe Rogers, user/survivor leader, stated:

> Twenty years ago we wouldn't have come out on the streets because we were afraid. We've been hidden away in closets and attics... Well, we're not going to be locked away any more... We're going to stand up and demand our rights as citizens.

Many have written about the downside of identifying as a user or survivor. For example:

> I have tremendous difficulty in seeing myself both as a competent researcher and as someone who has experienced mental health problems. Sometimes it is as though the two images of myself cannot co-exist: as one comes into focus, the other fades and becomes indistinct (Faulkner and Sayce 1997).

Yet increasing numbers are finding 'coming out' liberating (Connecticut Department of Health 1995), and not only on the streets:

> I've disclosed for political reasons. When I did this, I knew I was making myself vulnerable socially and professionally. But I figured the gains for other consumers and myself outweighed the risks. Identifying my disclosure and working with the larger civil rights movement has made it easier to run the risks of rejection or exclusion (service user).

It used to be the case that politicians did not survive if it were known that they had experienced any type of mental health problem. In 1971, Thomas Eagleton was dropped as vice-presidential candidate after it became known that he had had treatment for depression. In 1988, Ronald Reagan discredited his rival Michael Dukakis – also someone who had been treated for depression – by stating that he did not want to 'pick on an invalid'. By the 1990s, a change was in the air. When journalists got hold of the story in 1995 that Mrs Alma Powell was receiving treatment for depression, Colin Powell swiftly put an end to the story by confirming it: 'it is not a family secret,' he said, 'and I hope that people who read the story who think they might be suffering from depression make a beeline for the doctor, because it is something that can be dealt with very easily' (quoted in *Arizona Republic*, 9 November 1995). Journalists dropped the story, and Colin Powell's standing was undented. In 1998, when the Norwegian Prime Minister took time off with depression, 'Norwegians digested the news with sympathy', and even an arch political opponent applauded Mr Bondevik's decision to be open (*Independent*, 2 September 1998).

Some have been inspired by famous people who have come out. For example:

> I couldn't believe it when Princess Diana talked about her bulimia. I can't believe that I have something in common with her. I watched her and I thought, she's expected to perform as a princess and she can't do it. I have now talked to my family about my mental illness and they are proud of me (user/survivor, New Jersey, 1996).

We may be in the early stages of an unstoppable movement to refuse the shame of a diagnosis of mental illness. The eventual result could be that time off with depression, or manic depression, would go unremarked.

Creating shared understandings

User/survivors have raised consciousness through groups and writings, and have begun to articulate ideas that go against the grain of popular prejudice.

First, people have undermined the notion that mentally ill people are all 'the same', with the same experiences, not least by articulating the very different ways in which discrimination impinges on them. A large black man diagnosed with schizophrenia may see people cross the street to avoid him (Wilson 1997); while he is feared and demonised, an older white woman may rather be patronised as 'dotty' (Faulkner and Sayce 1997). A gay man may refuse to identify as a user because he remembers all too well when his sexuality rendered him mentally ill by definition; a lesbian user may be assumed to be 'mad' partly on the distinct grounds of non-conformity to a traditional woman's role (Sayce 1995c, Golding 1997). This is not an additive matter – of double or treble discrimination – but of being subjected to new, fused and potent stereotypes that are more than the sum of their parts. The 'black psycho-killer' image that repeatedly stares back from newspapers suggests that madness – and danger – have been located, by the white majority culture, in a group already seen as 'other', thus making them fit for intensified fear and hate. Joffe (1996) has shown how this process of 'anchoring' grave ills to the 'other' has occurred throughout history: syphilis was the French pox to the English, the *morbus Germanicus* to the Parisians and the Naples sickness to the Florentines (Sontag 1989). Similarly, people with AIDS were readily identified by majority cultures as black, gay or Haitian, thereby maintaining the construction of AIDS as 'not my group' (Joffe 1996).

User/survivors have begun to talk and write about difference: on cross-cutting grounds including gender, ethnicity, class, or type and degree of mental distress, for example:

> I thought the woman who believed the electrical equipment in her home was speaking to her was really mad. She thought that I was the really mad one because I used to scream from time to time (Faulkner and Sayce 1997).

Debate is increasing on the complex intersections of discrimination, on, for example, how men in the user movement can sometimes drown out women, arguing that their behaviour stems from distress (see, for example, Whittle 1998). Voices from some quarters – older people with mental health problems and user/survivors with physical or sensory impairments – are still relatively unheard. Gradually, however, differences are being unpicked between discrimination faced on visible grounds, such as ethnicity or many physical impairments, and on invisible grounds, which bring so many dilemmas about whether to 'pass' and when and how to 'come out' (Faulkner and Sayce 1997).

Second, users have progressively moved away from the argument that they should be accepted because they are just 'the same' as the wider society:

> Advocacy has really begun to take a hold. Martin Luther King showed us it was possible to be a gentleman and raise hell. Before I got involved in the consumer movement I couldn't reconcile mental illness and being a valid person. I can now [laughs]. I've moved from 'I haven't got this thing they say I've got – or if I have I'm not going to tell anyone

about it' – to maybe – maybe – it's OK to have it (user/survivor, Austin, Texas, 1996).

A packed 1997 British conference workshop on 'positive aspects of madness' elicited experiences including: profound spiritual understanding and joy, through visions; being able to write fiction, professionally, from the language received through voice hearing; new empathy, forged from the softened boundaries of psychosis, or from the depths of depression; an enhanced sensitivity to others; improved skills as a mental health worker; and finding community for the first time by moving from being a loner, rejected, to being part of the survivor movement (workshop originally devised by Read and Campbell 1995).

One man, when posed the question 'What would you do if someone called you a nutter?' replied, on video camera:

> I'd thank them for noticing. I am different. I'm proud of my differences – they're part of me.

People are turning the experience of madness over, revealing previously unseen sides. It is not irredeemably awful but mixed: at times tragic, wasteful, frustrating, boring, life denying; at other times, extraordinary in ways that contribute both to users' lives and to those around them. This revaluing of madness does not romanticise because it does not oust descriptions of terrors and trauma. It echoes the reclaiming of 'black', 'queer' and 'cripple' by other social movements.

Research on the upside of madness has most commonly focused on the links between creativity and manic depression. Jamison (1998) has shown that, during the highs, people asked to make word associations can make three times more associations, and three times more that are original, than people who are not 'manic'. For the imaginative and disciplined person, this rapid thought, punning and imagery of motion and colour – fire, waterfalls – becomes the stuff of poetry, painting or music. Meanwhile, mild melancholia can act as ballast, as editor – subduing or focusing thought, or transforming the experience of depression into new illuminations of the human condition. In addition, the transitions from high to low can leave people unusually at ease with ambiguities and with life 'on the edge'. These experiences may have underpinned work by artists from Samuel Johnson to Graham Greene. Far less is known of the potential advantages for activities from science to business, although personal accounts are beginning to reveal positive – as well as negative – experiences. Kay Jamison writes that she would not have missed her own experience of manic depression despite the times when she sits 'virtually inert, with a dead heart and a brain as cold as clay'. The highs, and the power to achieve, are unforgettable:

> The ideas and feelings are fast and furious like shooting stars... shyness goes, the right words are suddenly there, the power to captivate others a felt certainty (Jamison 1995).

Yet positive experiences do not appear to be exclusive to the diagnosis of manic depression. Peter Chadwick, a psychology lecturer diagnosed with schizophrenia, argues that psychosis can bring particular talents in the areas of creativity, social sensitivity and empathy (Chadwick 1997), and that the heightened awareness of others' motivations in paranoia may make people better able to distinguish between truth and lies:

> Sufferers of delusion do seem to be preoccupied at least at the time of the illness with issues of meaning and purpose. And it may be that psychosis can in a sense enhance a person's apprehension of their wider context of their place in the cosmic scheme of things... As I found myself, psychosis... can at least be the beginning of spiritual enlightenment. It may open doors to such experiences that the person can make productive use of later when they are well (*Independent*, 27 August 1997).

A wider public understanding of the positive side of madness seems likely as it is increasingly articulated by prominent, 'out' user/survivors. Actress Nicola Pagett states:

> Madness is not all flapping arms and dribbling. It is an altered state and, in a funny way, I wouldn't have missed it no matter how terrible it was... Remember that I have the drop on people. They don't know what it's like to go bananas. I quite like knowing about something that most people don't (*Guardian*, 27 August 1997).

'Mad' experiences can undoubtedly bring benefits to others. Melvyn Bragg has written eloquently of the impossibility of speaking, as a teenager, about his 'out of body' experiences:

I used to say my prayers then and yet I never mentioned this fear in them. For one thing, that would have been to extemporise, and the prayers I said were set ones, spoken twice on Sundays in church and most mornings in school assembly. There was no room for individual additions except to bless parents and relations... What was not allowed for was to tell anyone what was happening...

My parents could not have been better or kinder, but it was inconceivable that I could discuss this with them. How would I describe it? What would I, literally, say? (Bragg 1996).

His silence was not only attributable to a British formalism that allowed little individual expression. Until a language is created, people do not know what 'literally' to say. If all they hear is that having weird thoughts means you could be crazy, and that mentally ill people are hopeless and dangerous, they will probably say nothing. But when they hear or read of other people's strange experiences, it can enable them not only to speak of their own, but also to think them. Without a language, thought itself is silenced and truncated.

In 1998, the *Guardian* carried an article linking the slogan 'Glad to be mad' – which is how the Chair of Survivors Speak Out signed his letters – to the idea that the user movement 'could become Britain's next great movement for civil rights' (Freedland 1998).

A third point is that users have begun to articulate a model of 'social inclusion' that does not mean 'fitting in' and being accepted only if people 'pass' as 'normal', any more than wheelchair users should need to 'walk again' in order to be respected. It means including the experience of madness as part of our societies, valuing the people who experience it and recognising the contribution that madness can bring, as well as the pain it entails. As Shakespeare puts it in relation to disability generally:

Inclusion is different from integration. Integration implies the individual will fit in with the system: the person has to change. Inclusion means that the system itself will develop self-criticism; acknowledge the way in which it excludes and denies access; and dismantle barriers (Shakespeare 1997).

Rather than thinking of social inclusion in terms of a few excluded people moving from the periphery to the central area – as if British or American society had just one centre, one fixed

establishment – we need instead to think of an evolving landscape with many different 'peaks' where power resides. Inclusion
would mean both strengthening the power base of the
user/survivor movement and also ensuring that users had a fair
chance to move freely across the whole landscape, joining any
other power base they chose, from the environmental movement
to the political élite.

Fourth, users are beginning to chip away at the age-old idea that
the views of anyone who is 'mad' should, by definition, be discredited. As early as the 16th century, a patient in England, Nathaniel
Lee, reputedly highlighted the power imbalance that determines
whose views prevail:

> They called me mad, and I called them mad, and damn them they
> outvoted me (quoted in Porter 1991).

Most people experiencing even the full flood of 'madness' can be
'reliable witnesses'. They may hold certain beliefs – for example,
that they are being persecuted – that others around them do not
share or that are contradicted by other evidence, but these beliefs
do not permeate everything they experience and say. As Nicola
Pagett put it:

> Madness is very specific. When you think that the first piece of loo
> paper is poisoned, you also know that you have a relaxation class at half
> past two. So you know what a relaxation class is, and what half past two
> is (Brooks 1997).

Recognition of this specificity may in the future make it more
likely that users who report being assaulted will have the case
fully investigated – without being subjected to defence lawyers
insinuating that a psychiatric diagnosis per se discredits their
entire testimony (Home Office 1998).

Even where someone's specific thoughts would not stand up in a
court of law, they need not be invalidated: they have meaning for
the individual and they may also 'speak to' other people – witness,
for example, the interest in accounts of madness by writers such as
Janet Frame (Frame 1982). If the person's thoughts seem totally
inaccessible to others, their situation is likely to be extremely
isolated; they deserve respect and support. One woman told me of
the relief of eventually talking with someone else who had believed,
like her, that he was being pursued by people wanting to kill him.

This experience is as traumatic as actually being pursued but is not generally accorded the same weight or sympathy. As more user/survivors speak openly, and demonstrate that they have absorbing things to say, it will become harder to discredit users in general: the number of exceptions could stretch the credibility of the assumption that 'mentally ill' people are not worth listening to. This might create a little more room than at present to debate whose reality holds. Currently, people who are not 'mentally ill' define where the boundary lies between 'ill' and 'well'. Users could contribute to new thinking about madness and sanity, and about ways of making society fair for those deemed ill, mad, disabled or distressed.

Finally, users have begun to dent some of the most powerful myths about themselves. For example, among the majority of user/survivors who have never been violent, the constant assumption in the media (see Ch. 3), and in the minds of people they meet, that mental illness entails violence is painful and frustrating, and can lead to real discrimination. For example:

> My landlady said that when I first came to live in her house, there had been a programme on television about schizophrenia which had painted an extreme picture. The TV programme became a talking point with some acquaintances of hers and when my landlady announced that she had a schizophrenic lodger moving into her house they warned her against it. They worried that she might be murdered in her sleep... and that I was a walking time bomb (O'Donoghue 1994).

The actual association between violence and mental disorder is weak (Mullen *et al.* 1998, Steadman *et al.* 1998). One major study found that schizophrenia without the use of alcohol or drugs was not associated with raised rates of violent crime (although people with schizophrenia were more likely to use alcohol and drugs, and to be violent when they did) (Steadman *et al.* 1998). Others find a limited link between active psychosis and violence. An uncomfortable truth for the general public is that the vast majority of violent crime – over 95% in Britain – is committed by people who are *not* mentally ill. We cannot explain away the increase in violence by recourse to the concept of 'madness'. From 1957 to 1995, during the period of deinstitutionalisation, the proportion of homicides committed by people with a mental disorder actually fell steadily, from 35% to 11.5%, according to Home Office figures (Taylor and Gunn 1999). Factors that are more predictive than mental illness –

being young and male and the use of alcohol and drugs – receive far less fearful media attention than 'psycho-killer' stories, and there are no campaigns calling for the preventive detention of men who drink and assault their partners equivalent to those demanding the detention of mental patients. Curtailing user/survivors' rights always proves politically easier than with other, less powerless groups.

Some user/survivors do commit acts of violence. On occasion, the 'commonsense' view that this stems from their illness contains some truth, for example, if someone believes, as part of a delusion, that their only options are to fight someone or be killed themselves. Often, however, the violence is independent of the mental health problem: it arises from poverty, hopelessness, jealousy, gang battles between young men or other everyday situations (Sayce 1995a).

> Though she has never shown any violent tendencies, how can we be sure what might happen? In the back of my mind is the fear that one day she may harm someone physically (Meg Henderson, 1994, speaking of her daughter, diagnosed with a psychotic illness, *Guardian*, 20 August).

User/survivors are presumed guilty of potential violence – even if they have never been violent – and thus have virtually no way of proving themselves innocent. They have to challenge prevailing attitudes, from this unequal position, knowing that if they get angry, this may be seen as a confirmation of dangerous tendencies. This presents intense dilemmas in terms of how to present themselves – how, for example, to be effectively assertive at the same time as adopting a reasonable and demure style, in order to defuse the fear of madness.

User/survivors have adopted a range of useful strategies. They cite facts and comparisons:

> In all the three years that I have been going to the Psychiatric Day Hospital there have been no outbreaks of violence or trouble, unlike those I have seen in pubs (O'Donoghue 1994).

People also use humour:

> I've got my axe in my handbag (woman quoted in Sayce 1995a).

They also point out that they are more likely to be victims than offenders, a view increasingly being confirmed by research (Murphy 1991, Perkins and Repper 1998).

Those user/survivors who have been violent have articulated some of the sources of their anger, to break the assumption that their violence must be the result of raw madness. In a very rare media articulation of users/survivors' views, a 1996 British TV programme *The Merry-go-round*, screened around midnight, profiled two homeless people with mental health problems. Cas, a young woman, began her contradiction of dominant assumptions by explaining that she was the one at risk:

> People don't realise how vulnerable you are, specially when you're female. One of the things that I've had to do to get by is to shave my hair off and basically act a lot tougher than I am... Just because you're on the street doesn't mean you're not a person.

She went on to say, more unusually, that when she herself felt violent, it was not a disembodied symptom of illness:

> The DSS have just messed up yet again – which means I have to go out and humiliate myself totally by begging and get all the heat on the street as usual. I get so angry I can't even go in there. There's people daily arrested from this building. I get so angry and frustrated every time I even come near here I feel like bombing the place. That sounds really extreme but you wanna see the state of half the people who come out of here after they've been 'dealt with'.

Cas's account provides a counterblast to the usual discourse about users who are aggressive being 'thrown on the streets' without adequate controls, without forced medication. Cas's description does not lead viewers to that 'solution'. Rather, it illuminates different frustrations and possible resolutions: that women should have a safe place to sleep, that social security procedures should be made more fair and user-friendly, and that user/survivors should have improved support to help them with children if they lose their parental rights. All these have been the focus of user-led campaigns (Mind 1993, Sayce 1995b, Perkins and Foyster 1997).

The user/survivor movement may be poised to spread its understandings more widely and to secure a stronger foothold in society. User/survivors' experiences could then become an invaluable data source for policy makers. When Cas states that she can understand why 'so many people do go off their trolley' living on the streets, or when women describe the impact on their mental health of poverty, powerlessness and sexual assault, they provide information which could (in principle) lead policy makers to ask new questions of public health data, think creatively about primary prevention and set new trends in programme evaluation.

Numerous studies demonstrate links between unemployment, sexual abuse, poverty, poor housing, school exclusion, being brought up in care – and mental ill health (see, for example, Jahoda 1979, Huxley *et al.* 1989, Palmer *et al.* 1992, Henderson *et al.* 1998). Causation often goes in both directions. For example, unemployment and sexual assault leave people vulnerable to mental health problems (Mullen *et al.* 1988, Perkins and Silver 1994, Anthony *et al.* 1995, Link *et al.* 1997). In addition, mental health problems make unemployment more likely, and sexual assault more likely, because of employer rejection and because abusers know that their victims will not be believed if they report the crime (Read and Baker 1996, Home Office 1998). Preventive activities could be extended by adding a mental health dimension to cross-agency social inclusion initiatives – urban regeneration, Health Action Zones – so that community regeneration might effectively break into these interlocking patterns of discrimination and mental distress.

The aim is not to eliminate madness; given the mixed benefits and damage that it can bring (see above), the ethics of such an enterprise would be questionable. Attempts to wipe out schizophrenia or manic depression from the gene pool could leave society the poorer. But reducing the suffering of abuse, poverty and exclusion is desirable on humanitarian grounds. Policy makers could draw on user/survivors' experience in the effort to reduce social exclusion *per se*.

Conclusion

If we visualise a gradual move to a world where there is less discrimination towards, and less social exclusion of, people with mental health problems, the first staging post would be a place where people are listening to what those 'on the edge' are saying. Those who are not user/survivors would no longer rely on stereotypes *about* people with mental health problems put over by other people. The 'hole' in the public discussion would be filled, by a range of different experiences and analyses from user/survivors.

For the next stage of development – beyond 'community care' services to opportunities to contribute and be included in society – we need a new set of fantasies, which will become the reality of the 21st century, just as user-run services were developed in the 1980s from the dreams of the 1970s. To have power, users' and allies' voices need to reach further beyond the circle of survivors and mental health professionals to wider public and decision-making audiences.

The black civil rights dream enabled millions of people to imagine that the world could be otherwise. For example:

> My father muses: 'It's funny... we talked about race all the time, yet at the same time you never really thought about *how* it could be different. But after *Brown* I remember it dawning on me that I *could* have gone to the University of Georgia. And people started to talk to you a little differently; I remember [the white doctor] used to treat us in such a completely offhand way. But after *Brown*, he wanted to discuss it with us, he asked questions, what I thought. He wanted my opinion and I suddenly realised that no white person had ever asked what I thought about anything' (Williams P. 1995).

In the mental health world, we need to imagine that things that seem inevitable could be different.

We also need to acknowledge the fact that the growth in social exclusion seen over the past two decades shows no immediate sign of abating, government intentions notwithstanding (Lister 1997). This may not be a climate in which the voice of 'mad' people who are excluded will hold its audience. Policy makers may have little to gain from listening to people who can tell them about the results of patterned experiences such as the widespread assault of women and children, or increasing relative poverty, or the exclusion of black children from schools. Until government and a wide range of social institutions begin to reduce inequality and social exclusion, the voices of people on the margins are likely to remain unheard.

In pursuing dreams of social inclusion and access, we need to recognise that there could be a very different future in store – one in which social exclusion becomes ever more pronounced for some groups and individuals, and ever more inescapable for people with a diagnosis of serious mental illness.

CHAPTER 2

Future Dreams,
Future Nightmares

The growth of inequality

It's like being hidden. It's as if you have been put in a garage where, if
they don't have room for something but aren't sure if they should throw
it out, they put it there, where they don't need to think of it again... If
people in New York woke up one day and learned that we were gone,
that we had simply died or left for somewhere else, how would they
feel? I think they'd be relieved... People in Manhattan could go on and
lead their lives and not feel worried about being robbed and not feel
guilty and not need to pay for welfare babies... I think they look on us
as obstacles to moving forward (15-year-old girl living on the New York
streets, quoted in Kozol 1995).

Far from harnessing the ideas and experiences of people on the social
margins to inform social change, we may find that their number
continues to grow and that the public demands an ever firmer
management of the visible poor, and makes increasingly strenuous
efforts to avoid them.

In what Chomsky has termed the 'thirdworldization' of the US
(Chomsky 1994), polarities of wealth and poverty – long established between so-called 'first' and 'third' world countries – are
beginning to be repeated within the single country of the US. In
1996, the Agency for International Development – a branch of the
US Government – decided to go into Southeast Washington DC,
where it found conditions to be 'depressingly similar to those in the
third world' (*Washington Post*, 11 February 1996). In the mid-1990s,
this capital city had an average salary for those employed ($40,919)
that was over 50% higher than the national average; it also had a

higher poverty rate (21%) than any state other than Louisiana (Vedder 1996).

Specific geographical areas – Anacostia in Washington, the South side of Chicago – and particular segments of society within them, for example, African American men in Harlem, suffer extreme forms of social exclusion, ill-health and violent crime. Louisiana and Mississippi, with the highest income disparities, top the list for deaths per 100,000 and for homicides per 100,000 (Wilkinson 1996). For boys born in Harlem, life expectancy is lower than for boys born in Bangladesh (McCord and Freeman 1990). For black people in the US generally, life expectancy is not only at least 6 years lower than for whites, but also began to fall in the mid-1980s, while for whites it continued to rise (Wilkinson 1996). In 1978, an average director of a large US company earned about 60 times the earnings of a typical worker; by 1995 she or he earned about 170 times as much (Cassidy 1997).

In Britain, economic inequality is not as extreme as in the US but has since 1985 grown slightly faster (Wilkinson 1996). From 1979 to 1993/94, the number living below half-average household income (after housing costs) – that is, below the generally accepted poverty line – rose from 5 million to 13.7 million, that is, from 9% to 22% of the population. Income after housing costs fell for the bottom decile by 13% and rose for the top decile by 65% (Lister 1997).

As in the US, the problem of highly specific segments of population experiencing exclusion is growing. In 1997, the British government identified a 'threat of growing inequality – stemming from the risk that globalisation and uneven access to new technologies could widen the gap between the successful and the least skilled, the well-off and the socially excluded, unless headed off by strong government action' (Department for Education and Employment 1997). Social exclusion was seen to apply not only to the officially unemployed, but also to more specific sub-groups, for example to 150,000 homeless people, to jobless ethnic minority communities, to women out of work for lack of childcare and to people excluded because of disability. In some parts of the country, such as some inner city areas and run-down housing estates, 'economic, educational and social deprivation have spanned several generations'.

Architect Richard Rogers has described how growing inequality, and the fear of crime that it generates, have visibly changed the geography of American cities:

Our public spaces are seen as downright dangerous... The street market becomes less attractive than the secured shopping mall, the university district becomes the closed campus; and as this process spreads through the city the open-minded public domain retreats. People with wealth bar themselves in or move out of the city. In these closed, privatised spaces, the poor are forbidden to enter, guards stand at the gate. Those without money are equivalent to those without a passport, a class to be banished... We created cities to celebrate what we have in common. Now they are designed to keep us apart (Rogers 1997).

Over 30 million Americans live in gated communities, typically guarded by armed security. The same pattern occurs in European cities 'writ small' (Rogers 1997).

'Managing' the poor can take harsh forms. In Atlanta, Georgia, some of the streets have trees in them with a small wall surrounding each. Spikes have been added to the walls to stop homeless people sitting on them. Davis (1992) describes how, in Los Angeles, 'one popular seafood restaurant has spent $12,000 to build the ultimate bag-lady proof trash cage: made of three-quarter-inch steel rod with alloy locks and vicious outturned spikes to safeguard priceless mouldering fishheads and stale french fries' (quoted in P Williams 1995).

As crime (in some areas) and fear of crime have increased in parallel with relative poverty, ever harsher responses have been instigated, alongside attempts to prevent crime. The US has the second highest rate of imprisonment in the world, with 1.8 million prisoners in 1999, and Britain the highest rate in Europe. Large numbers of inmates come from the very situations of extreme relative poverty described above. In the US, by the mid-1990s, one-third of black men in their twenties were either in jail or under the supervision of the criminal justice system. Executions also increased. The 1994 Crime Bill provided for the death penalty for 60 federal offences. In Georgia, figures showed that a black person was 11 times more likely to be executed for murder of a white person than was a white person for murder of someone black (Bright 1995).

The public is influenced in its demand for tough action on crime by exaggerated beliefs about its frequency. The 1997 British Crime Survey found that people overestimated the number of crimes committed and massively underestimated the severity of punishments already given. Their fears had grown over the previous decade. News reporting of 'bad' news, soap operas (which include far more tragic events per episode than is statistically likely) and TV crime shows all appeared to fuel the concerns. In addition, as visible poverty increases, public helplessness turns easily to 'individual failure' explanations, which justify fear of the poor and punitive treatment. In this climate victims' organisations have a growing influence: for example, in Britain, released sex offenders who have served their sentences have increasingly faced public demonstrations and have in some cases been hounded from town to town. Rules on release have been tightened.

Far from marginalised groups working together to counteract intersecting discriminations and achieve inclusion (see Ch. 1), they may find that they are increasingly excluded and disproportionately punished. They may continue to be subjected to increasing numbers of targeted hate crimes (P Williams 1995). They could find that 'talk radio' and the Internet provide ever more space where there are no constraints on the expression of bigotry, where hate on the airwaves is 'exalted as freedom' and a mass market of white, male, middle-class Americans is addressed 'as an endangered minority' (P Williams 1995).

The impact of inequality on users of mental health services

Increasing social inequality, crime, fear of crime and related trends impact on people with mental health problems both because social exclusion itself creates distress and because those who are disadvantaged by the social status of the 'mental patient' become caught up in punitive, excluding policies and public moods.

People with mental health problems – at a major disadvantage in the labour market (see Ch. 3) – are at high risk of poverty, ill-health, homelessness and imprisonment. In 1995, America's jails held over 640,000 people with severe mental illness. Typically, in American cities, those running mental health services report that social exclusion has intensified for people with severe mental health problems, sometimes even where mental health services have improved. In San Francisco from 1990–95, mental health budgets remained stable or even increased slightly. The ratio of hospital to community services changed from 90:10, to 60:40 so that users could be offered ongoing support in the context of their ordinary lives. Yet enlightened mental health policies were powerless to stem the trend of the increased marginalisation of users, which resulted from the general increase in incarceration and the decline in affordable housing. Dr

Okin, Chief of Psychiatry at San Francisco General Hospital, notes that discriminatory attitudes on the part of the public worsen in these circumstances. As more people with mental health problems live on the streets, the public's image of someone with mental illness comes to be a person who is begging, who acts strangely – and who is a threat (Okin, personal communication, 1996).

Moreover, the public fear of crime becomes channelled into the fear of specific groups – mentally ill people, homeless people, people who take drugs, black people. In Britain, the scapegoating of user/survivors in the media in the 1990s was intense, with an endless stream of media stories about 'crazed killers' (Philo et al. 1993). A few highly atypical cases of homicide committed against strangers became emblematic of public fear (Sayce 1995a). In fact, most homicides committed by user/survivors, as with homicides generally, target known victims, often family members (Boyd 1994).

Users suffer from this scapegoating not only because the imagery is frightening and distressing (see Ch. 1), but also because the 'moral panic' appears to be linked to growing hostility in the 1990s towards mental health facilities and the people who use them (Sayce 1998a). Repeated Department of Health public opinion surveys have shown an increasing minority expressing a fear of mentally ill people: in 1993, 14% of a representative sample of 2000 adults thought it was frightening to think of people with mental health problems living in residential neighbourhoods; this figure had risen to 19% by 1996 and to 25% by 1997 (Department of Health 1993, 1997).

Repper et al. (1997) found that over two-thirds of mental health service providers surveyed, in both the statutory and voluntary sectors, had experienced increased 'nimby' opposition from 1992 to 1997. Sixty-three per cent of voluntary Mind associations had had to delay a development because of opposition and 30% had withdrawn plans altogether. In some 'nimby' campaigns, neighbours have liter-ally demanded that high fences be built all round small supported housing projects (Professor Tom Craig, personal communication, 1997). In South London, the following slogan appeared painted on a van in a street where a mental health service was to open:

'Schizophrenics go home'

This was ironic given that people were actually trying to set up home but were prevented from doing so by neighbours who appeared to believe that service users belonged somewhere else –

preferably in a distant institution. They were not seen as part of the local community.

The research suggests that those who appear to face the worst 'nimby' opposition in Britain are young black men (Repper *et al.* 1997); in this case, the phrase 'go home' has a parallel, racist set of associations. It appears that some predominantly white British communities wish to exclude black people and the 'mad', both of whom, they think, may cause violence, change the tenor of the neighbourhood and bring house prices down.

These rejections can impact further on people's mental health:

> The feeling that the community doesn't like them has led to deterioration in some people's mental health (local Mind association, quoted in Repper *et al.* 1997).

Worsened distress can render people more obvious targets for attack or verbal harassment (see Ch. 3) , which can in turn increase distress in a potentially endless vicious circle.

As in the broader criminal justice sector, victims' rights are taking precedence over users' rights in public and political debate. In Britain, an organisation representing victims of mentally disordered offenders – the Zito Trust – achieved widespread publicity by arguing (inaccurately) that violence committed by user/survivors had risen as a result of community care failures. 'In cases where someone who commits a crime has been deemed to be mentally ill the victims of crime are still victims: but in their case they have absolutely no rights' (Zito Trust 1997). In 1998, the government responded to these concerns by stating, despite extensive evidence to the contrary (see Ch. 1), that 'care in the community has failed'. The Minister argued that patients had been 'left to become a danger to themselves and a nuisance to others' (Dobson 1998) and that the first priority of mental health services was public safety. These pronouncements reinforced public misconceptions, being quoted in later 'nimby' campaigns, and caused consternation among user/survivors, who called helplines in considerable numbers to express their fears of being reinstitutionalised. The government did not take the opportunity to articulate a vision of inclusion for user/survivors alongside other disabled people, despite social inclusion being the hallmark of its policy of the moment.

If governments, in the UK, the US and elsewhere, fail to 'head off' increased social exclusion – to 'break these patterns of deprivation, the dead weight of low expectation and the crushing belief that things cannot get better', as the British Department of Education and Employment put it in 1997 – we could see an increasing number of hate crimes against service users and ever more damaging effects of marginalisation, especially for people facing discrimination on several fronts (those who are service users, and black, and drug users). This raises the critical question, are governments likely to succeed?

Measures to reduce social exclusion

In late 1997, Tony Blair announced measures aiming to improve life for an estimated 5 million Britons affected by crime, unemployment, ignorance and bad housing:

> We are passionately committed to making Britain one nation, giving every single person a stake in the future and tackling chronic poverty and social division (Tony Blair, quoted in *Independent on Sunday*, 7 December 1997).

The way proposed to achieve this was to enhance responsibilities rather than just rights and to strengthen the ties of family and community. For example, New Labour was 'reforming the welfare state around the work ethic': all who were capable of working had a responsibility to do so (speech by Secretary of State for Social Security to the Labour Party Conference October 1997, *Guardian*, 14 November 1997). This view, broadly supported by the Conservative opposition, represented a new political consensus – the third of the post-war era.

In the 1940s, political parties united over the need for universal welfare state entitlements. The 1942 Beveridge Report promised an end to the 'poor law' policy of deterring idleness through keeping payments to the old, the sick and the unemployed to a minimum. It promised instead a universal social insurance system that would provide subsistence for all, with no means test, an end to mass unemployment and a national health service.

By the 1970s, this aim of universalism had been eroded. Unemployment was higher than expected, universal benefits too costly and social security benefits means-tested in ever more complex ways.

In the 1990s, the third consensus view – which had emerged earlier in the US – was that the receipt of welfare state benefits should be neither universal, nor just means-tested, but distributed according to moral behaviour. In order to receive benefits, one had actively to seek work, desist from taking drugs and otherwise behave responsibly.

Welfare state entitlement was no longer seen as the means of reducing poverty and inequality. Instead, social exclusion would be remedied through reducing dependency on the welfare state. Dependency on welfare, rather than poverty or inequality *per se*, began to be seen as the root of social exclusion. Decades of social programmes, which had created this dependency, were deemed by many commentators to have failed. Thus, in 1992, a Democratic President, supported by Republican colleagues, called for an 'end to welfare as we know it', and in 1997, a British Labour government (supported by Conservatives) echoed American rhetoric to the word, proposing a 'hand-up not a hand-out', 'welfare-to-work', and 'an end to the dependency culture'.

In many ways, this shift from the ideal of universalism to means-testing, to a morally based allocation of welfare, is a mirror image of the earlier change from the Victorian Poor Law – which allocated help to the 'deserving' but not the 'undeserving' poor – to the means tests of the 1930s and then to the hope of universalism of the 1940s. The particular 'progress' of the second half of the 20th century could be viewed as a simple reversal of what was seen as 'progress' in the first half.

There are major differences between the American and British 'welfare state' systems. The US has no long-term unemployment benefit for single people. It never developed a national health service, and in 1997, it had over 30 million citizens with no public or private health care coverage at all (*Economist*, 15 December 1997). There is nothing in Britain to compare to the phenomenon of Americans travelling to a much poorer country – Mexico – to obtain health services at affordable prices. In the border towns, stalls filled with Mexican souvenirs vie for shoppers' attention with strings of discount pharmacies, dentists and physicians' offices, all offering products far more cheaply than in the US.

Yet American rhetoric, and some American policies, have influenced developments in Britain. Prior to the mid-1990s, the British did not use the term 'welfare' to mean income maintenance; instead, they talked of social security or income support. Seemingly in the interests of highlighting the difference between a positive (the 'work' ethic) and a negative, they picked a term 'welfare', which the Americans had already imbued with imagery of hopelessness. Policy initiatives from welfare-to-work schemes to the creation of a 'drugs czar' also carried echoes of previous American developments, although they were moulded to fit goals of social inclusion rather than individual self-reliance alone.

History will determine whether morally based social policy will be effective in reducing chronic poverty, social division and the mental health problems, crime and other social ills that they can exacerbate. The moral expectation that young people will contribute to society could lift many out of hopelessness. Several commentators have, however, argued that welfare-to-work schemes cannot succeed without economic policies that increase job availability, especially in geographical pockets of extremely high unemployment (Hutton 1997, Donnison 1998, Social Policy Association 1998). In the US, where many states have lifetime limits on the receipt of welfare of 2 or 3 years, destitution or dependency on church or charity can follow. Julius Wilson argued that in New York in 1996/97 there were 50,000 job vacancies, yet 300,000 people were out of work and in many cases not eligible for welfare or food stamps (Franklin 1997). The problem with the 'new moralist' welfare agenda may be not the moral emphasis *per se* but the balance of responsibilities:

> With all the duties of individual benefit recipients to take up work and training opportunities, where... is the duty on government and employers to provide such opportunities? (Social Policy Association 1998).

Policies requiring reduced dependency on the state can mean an increased dependency on other family members. This can exacerbate power imbalances between women and men, or disabled people and those who support them. P Williams (1995) argues that workfare has been supplemented by bridefare – women are expected to work or to marry in order 'to receive some measure of what they need'.

In Britain, in 1997, a group of 54 professors of social policy criticised the government's approach to reducing exclusion because it 'erased from the map' the issue of income redistribution. The government replied that the main path out of social exclusion was the mainstream economy – 'with its opportunities and risks' (*Guardian*, 14 November 1997). The critics noted that risks, by their nature, mean that some people lose.

The criticisms were put more bluntly by American demonstrators against the 1996 Welfare Act. Activists from the National Organisation of Women, the Rainbow Coalition and many children's, minority and disability groups argued that the aim should be not to 'end welfare as we know it', as Clinton had promised, but to 'end poverty as we know it'. These critics saw the new consensus bleakly: to them, both democrat and republican, Clinton and Gingrich, were abandoning the poor.

Evaluations of welfare-to-work schemes – like the internationally heralded programme in Riverside, California, cited in Britain by both main political parties in their 1997 manifestos – had not by the late 1990s demonstrated a long-term success in altering labour market participation, although they did suggest a short-term success in reducing the number of welfare recipients (Peck 1996). The British Government, in particular, also invested in the late 1990s in a range of initiatives to revitalise communities, enhance educational attainment, reduce crime and improve health and inclusion through inter-agency co-ordination and community participation. Evaluations of such initiatives will be critical to future policy planning.

Implications for users of mental health services

For mental health service users, the new emphasis on responsibilities as well as rights could have major benefits. Users have been denied the chance to contribute, to take responsibility, on a massive scale (see Ch. 3). The idea of 'responsibility' holds out the hope of being able to work, to raise children – to be full citizens for the first time. It could mean, in principle, that users would be expected to take total, or in some cases partial, responsibility for crimes they committed, like other citizens and would, as a corollary, be given finite sentences rather than an incarceration of uncertain duration. In addition, they would no longer be subject to preventive detention on a different basis from other citizens.

It does seem likely that welfare-to-work initiatives will enable some service users to gain work and in some cases to keep it. This could be transformative. However, the impact of social inclusion measures generally will depend enormously on who defines responsibility and how. Here, there are risks for service users.

First, new responsibilities are not simply being matched to existing rights: in some cases, individual rights are being reduced at the same time as individual responsibilities are increased. For example, in the US, the 1996 Personal Responsibility and Work Opportunity Reconciliation Act (generally known as the Welfare

Act; see above) effectively abolished any entitlement under federal law to welfare. The responsibility for setting criteria was passed to individual states, and even at state level, individuals had no legal right to challenge the criteria, nor how they were applied. Thus, the nation backed out of any social responsibility to protect vulnerable people from poverty, simultaneously expecting individuals to take on more responsibility in terms of seeking work and not taking drugs (see below).

The US devolved more and more decisions on eligibility to public services to the states – for Medicaid, housing, social security – at the same time as significantly reducing budgets. The 'entitlement society' had ended, and with it many pre-existing collective responsibilities. This is a more major shift than simply 'correcting' an imbalance between responsibilities and rights.

In future Britain, as well as the US, pressures to reduce disability benefit expenditure could mean that some disabled people would lose benefits because they were deemed capable of work, of taking responsibility, but would still not be able to find work because discrimination by employers would not have been dismantled nor access ensured. The trend in the employment of disabled people since the 1970s has been downward; as the supply of labour has overtaken demand, employers have become more selective (Berthoud 1998). In this case, the rhetoric of individual responsibility could lead to a net loss of income, and increased social exclusion, at least for some people with mental health problems. Hills (1998) argues that we could see a 'race' between the positive impact of policy measures to increase work opportunities and the negative effects of falling relative income for those remaining on benefits (Hills 1998).

Second, in order to receive benefits such as public housing, one has to behave responsibly. In both the US and the UK, measures have been introduced to ensure that people who behave in antisocial ways can be evicted from public housing. But who decides what 'antisocial' behaviour is? When, for example, someone is talking to himself and his neighbour hounds him for being a 'nutter' – which can sometimes take vicious forms – which person gets evicted? British government rhetoric at times supports the idea that people with mental health problems can be a nuisance and a danger, thus potentially legitimising neighbours' views that they should not have to put up with 'crazy' people living next door. Neighbours may think that the first approach should be eviction or institutionalisation rather than problem solving, putting in extra support for the user or challenging prejudices.

While major noise and risk must be challenged – and users should not be excused for bad behaviour – there is a risk that simply 'odd' behaviour will be less tolerated, even when it is not damaging or dangerous. The mantra of responsibility could become a simple cloak for prejudice.

In the US in the mid-1990s, the rights of disabled children to integrated education came under attack. Some politicians made a strong case for defining behavioural and emotional disturbance as bad behaviour rather than disability, thereby excluding such children from school. They questioned who should 'really be in our schools', as a member of Newt Gingrich's Task Force on the issue put it in 1995. Someone with emotional difficulties was evidently not seen as one of 'us', with rights to attend 'our' schools. The consequence, if such views prevailed, could be loss of education for children with multiple emotional and social difficulties – with all the risk of later unemployment, crime and mental health problems that this would entail.

Instead of communities being asked to adapt, to improve access for people with mental health problems – as advocated in Chapter 1 – this approach asks children or adults with mental health problems to fit in to society as it is or lose housing, education and other basic requirements.

The risks of increased exclusion are particularly evident in relation to people who take illegal drugs. In the US in 1996, fuelled by the national 'war on drugs', Clinton announced that federal resources to the states for public housing would be weighted in favour of states that promptly evicted tenants accused (not even convicted) of a crime. Much of the public and political debate centred on drug offences. Faced with criticism from civil rights groups – who pointed out that this was a 'no strikes and you're out' policy, as it did not require even a single conviction – the Secretary of the Housing and Urban Development Department (HUD) stated that there was only money for about a quarter of those eligible for public housing and that it was therefore only reasonable for authorities to show a strong intolerance of tenants who caused problems. Public housing 'is a privilege', he stated, thereby clearly exemplifying the end of the entitlement era in favour of demonstrating one's 'deserving' status. Authorities who did not evict people risked losing money and potentially having their management taken over by HUD (as happened in Washington DC) (*Washington Post*, 29 March 1996).

Also in 1996, the Social Security Administration wrote to about 250,000 people receiving disability benefits on the basis of an addiction problem, informing them that their benefit was terminated. Alcohol and drug problems ceased to count as a disability for the purposes of the 'SSI' disability benefit. Spouses and children lost their benefit too.

Also in 1996, the Personal Responsibility and Work Opportunity Reconciliation Act brought in punitive restrictions for people who used drugs. Anyone convicted of a drug felony, including drug use, possession or distribution, after 22 August 1996 lost entitlement to welfare cash benefits and food stamps *permanently*. Anyone who violated their probation or parole conditions also became ineligible for welfare cash or food stamps, and welfare recipients generally could be drug-tested – and lose welfare if they tested positive.

The poverty and homelessness that these measures can create for drug users, many of whom have no Medicaid entitlement and no access to treatment for addiction problems, can lead people almost inexorably into crime in order to eat and/or to pay for the drugs to which they are often addicted. If jailed, people are released to a situation of zero welfare or food, often little chance to work and precious little motivation to make a new start in life. People who have nothing to lose may become still more prone to crime. It is highly questionable whether these risks are outweighed by the possible deterrent effect of punitive policies. These policies impact heavily on people with concurrent drug and mental health problems (Sayce 1997b).

If a country wants people to take responsibility by, for example, not committing drug offences, it might at the least take responsibility itself for ensuring that treatment, food, housing and the chance to work are on offer for those agreeing to be rehabilitated. Numerous studies suggest that this approach would be more cost-effective than only policing drug supply and punishing drug users (Sayce 1997b). It might further question whether it is a fair balance of rights and responsibilities to remove all the basics of life after a prison sentence has been served, in response to someone committing a single crime.

In Britain, the new emphasis on responsibility is in part balanced by new rights. For example, the 1998 incorporation of the European Convention on Human Rights (which takes Britain nearer to an equivalent of the American Bill of Rights) enables service users to challenge the infringement of their rights to privacy, liberty and the like in British courts. Also, traditions of social responsibility are stronger than in the US. For example, Britain invested £217 million in drug treatment services in 1998. However, the debate about rights and responsibility in both countries has become excessively divorced from discussions of power. It is those with power, not those with rights, who most critically need to take responsibility for their actions.

It is commonly stated on both sides of the Atlantic that rights and responsibilities have got out of balance: welfare recipients demand rights but do not take responsibility for remedying their situation. Similarly, in the mental health world, service users want the right to refuse treatment but do not always want to take equal responsibility with other citizens for working or facing the consequences of crimes (see Ch. 6). In the current policy climate, with its vehement emphasis on individual responsibility (especially in the US), this is not the most significant imbalance. It is rather the imbalance between the responsibility expected of individuals, particularly very powerless individuals, and that expected of groups and whole societies.

Although some policies have emerged that are designed to change the social environment so that disabled people can participate, there is a very strong policy push for everyone – emotionally disturbed children in schools or people taking drugs on housing estates – to change themselves to fit in with the social norm. They have to take responsibility, even if society shows little responsibility, or flexibility, in accommodating them. The way in which responsibility is defined is determined by social norms that are created by people who have power. Thus men, backed by some women, may decide that women are irresponsible if they choose to have children out of wedlock, and 'sane' people decide that 'mad' people should not act strangely on housing estates or underground trains (even if they do no harm). Powerful people determine that those who steal when they have no more access to food stamps should be punished, rather than considering the responsibility of a whole society to avoid placing people in that position in the first place.

At worst, 'responsibility' is used to blame powerless people for social problems. For example, according to P Williams (1995), the subliminal suggestion in the US media that black women 'have no business having any more children' is part of a welfare war in which the enemy is not poverty but poor people. Similarly, the war on drugs may become the war on drug users (Sayce 1997b).

Culturally, 'shame' is back in fashion. Etzioni argued in 1997 that stigma was a humane force (*Observer*, 13 July 1997). The risk of emphasising responsibility and shame is that users will be made to feel ashamed for being different or for being unable to take full responsibility all the time. They have enough shame to contend with without it being deliberately fostered.

If this imbalance in the discussion of rights and responsibilities continues, the future may be one in which people who do not fit the dominant views of what it means to take responsibility will find themselves ever more marginalised.

Strengthening 'community'

The so-called 'breakdown' of community has spawned many attempts deliberately to foster community spirit. However, it is questionable whether 'community' has broken down. For many people, it is rather that geographical community has been replaced by dispersed communities of interest.

But where groups – geographical, religious and political – are responding to concern about supposed 'breakdown', they tend to make deliberate attempts to bolster their own sense of identity and belonging. This often means hardening the group's edges. We know who belongs by defining who is excluded. People with mental health problems usually find themselves on the wrong side of the line. They may even, by being so clearly 'other' and unwanted, help to define who is included,

For example, writers on the new urbanism advocate replacing sprawling suburbs with neighbourhoods measuring a quarter of a mile from centre to edge (Katz 1995). These are precisely the types of community which, in the US, appear most likely to generate 'nimby' campaigns and other rejections of people with mental health problems. Although British research finds 'nimbyism' to be as common in poorer areas as in richer (Repper *et al.* 1997), American research suggests that it is strongest in areas with powerful individual advocates and a collective organisation such as a strong neighbourhood association (Robert Wood Johnson Foundation 1990). Areas with a strong identity and community organisation may thus be harsher environments for user/survivors than more amorphous, anonymous areas.

Some minority groups – ethnic, religious and sexual – also promote their sense of 'community' in ways that may exclude people with mental health problems. For example, the Million Man March of 1995, and its British counterpart in 1998, emphasised creating community through personal responsibility and encouraged hundreds of thousands of black men to aspire to a life less dominated by incarceration and poverty. Men should take responsibility for their families and communities, women for their specific family role. For people with mental health problems, these relatively traditional definitions can be problematic: their mental health difficulties may have partly stemmed from some of these traditional roles, for example abuses of power within a family (Palmer *et al.* 1992, Perkins *et al.* 1996). Also, once using mental health services, they may be unable to fulfil the roles required: a man, for instance, may be unable to secure work and be a breadwinner.

The injunction to act strong is common in minority communities; those which are trying to present themselves as successful have a vested interest in denying the presence of 'madness' in their midst. For example, until recently, many Hispanic Americans in Southern Texas literally kept disabled family members hidden (Perez 1994).

Gay men and lesbians wish to deny 'madness' because of having been so recently seen as mentally ill by definition; indeed, some psychoanalysts still offer reparative therapy (Sayce 1995c). Now the aim is to be out and proud – and definitively not 'sick'. While, in some circles, mental health service users are accommodated – the Michigan Women's Music Festival, for example, began to provide mental health support following an outcry when a woman was removed from the festival and forcibly detained in hospital – many people still dare not 'come out' as lesbian or gay in the user/survivor movement, nor as a user in gay circles. This is ironic given the depth of both communities' understandings of the dilemmas of 'coming out' (Sayce 1995c).

As communities try to strengthen themselves, they often revert to traditional beliefs rather than forge new ground. For users, this means that they can often join as long as they assimilate and act 'normal'. As one user put it with reference to involvement in his local church, 'they say everyone is welcome, but when you act a bit different, or have a mannerism that's a bit peculiar, they don't want you' (user/survivor, Alabama, 1996). Traditionally, Christianity holds that sin and the devil are the origin of most psychosis; to abandon this notion would be 'a challenge to the New Testament itself' (Dain 1992). In some fundamentalist groups, users can participate at the cost of seeing their mental health problems as a sin. This notion is also commonplace in widely available Christian self-help books. One on sale in 1996 concluded with a chapter entitled 'Confess your depression' (to God). 'I realized I had carried my depression too far... I confessed, admitted and agreed that my depression was a sin, something not in accordance with God's will for my life. I then asked God to forgive me for being gloomy and unproductive for so long' (Littauer 1986). One Catholic 12-step book shows how the angels can be brought into the process of confession (Taylor 1992). While many churches offer real chances of inclusion for user/survivors, the more fundamentalist teachings tend to the view that people should be ashamed of being mentally ill.

There are communities – for example, the movement for inclusion in education – that aim to create a new sense of community, based on including everyone: 'we're all born in', as one advocate of inclusion put it (Bates 1997). But these exceptions prove the rule. In some ways, user/survivors may have as much to fear from a new emphasis on strong 'communities' as they do from the supposed 'breakdown' of community.

Conclusion: dream or nightmare?

The 'real' future is not predetermined. One futurologist who has ventured a view – Arthur C Clarke – invents a fictional character who is 'surprised' to find lunatic asylums still operating in 3001. He describes how technical methods have also been found of detecting impending psychosis so that those affected can be controlled through a 'brain cap'. Civil liberties concerns – articulated in the slogan 'brain cap or brain cop?' – quickly gave way to the realisation that strong control was necessary to prevent the greater evil of terrorist activities by fanatical, especially religious, groups (Clarke 1997).

In the nearer future, it is possible that inequality, intolerance, exclusion and coercion could compound each other in a series of vicious circles: the faster the growth of inequality, the more the need for scapegoats; the greater the social exclusion, the worse the mental health problems; the stranger the behaviour, the greater the intolerance. Coercion could spread – from institutions right through community settings – with user/survivors' voices ever more eclipsed, their content explained through biodeterminism. New fault lines might emerge in the user movement over where to compromise.

Yet, in the US in the 1980s, disabled people achieved greatly enhanced rights at a time when homelessness and unemployment were devastating the lives of many, including disabled people. At the turn of the century, it is realistic to aim for improved civil rights law and a reduction in stereotyped media coverage. Where progress is blocked – as when the fear of crime and disorder is so high that explanations in terms of madness are hard to dislodge – energies can be expended on developing and sharing ideas to prepare for more favourable conditions.

Attacks on users' interests could also provide a jolt to action, just as saturation media coverage of homicides in 1990s Britain prompted organisations ranging from the Health Education Authority to the Royal College of Psychiatrists to tackle 'stigma'. The policy debate on rights and responsibilities presents major new opportunities, as well as risks, and users may succeed in moulding initiatives such as welfare-to-work to fit their own interests.

Yet if, over the next 20 years, inequality in general were to be effectively reduced, this would not in itself create inclusion for users. Discrimination on mental health grounds intersects with discrimination on grounds such as income, gender and ethnicity but is not reducible to them. The discrimination faced by people who are seen as 'imperfect' – those who are not 'body beautiful' and those deemed mentally 'imperfect, dangerous and unreliable' – must be challenged head on.

To achieve social inclusion in a highly complex and changing environment requires alliances to address those risks of exclusion which are shared (between homeless people, disabled people and different minority ethnic communities) and to ensure that neither policy makers nor their allies pursue 'inclusion' to the 'exclusion' of mental health service users. The rest of this book is a contribution to the analysis of how to achieve this, beginning in Ch. 3 with an examination of the legacy and impact of mental health discrimination on user/survivors.

CHAPTER 3

The Illusion of Citizenship

Equal citizens?

The fact that people with mental health problems may not be full citizens – sharing rights, responsibilities and complete membership of a society with everyone else – is evident in some countries at the point of entry.

For foreigners arriving in the US, the visa waiver arrival forms begin promisingly with the words 'welcome to the United States'. They go on to enquire whether a list of ills including the following apply to you: moral turpitude, prior engagement in espionage, terrorist activities, genocide – or mental disorder (US Department of Justice 1-94W Non-immigrant visa waiver arrival/departure form). Although Immigration and Naturalization Service (INS) officials state, when asked, that having a mental disorder is not always a bar to entry, there is no hint of this on the forms. For immigrant visas, 'mental disorder' is used as a filter for screening for possible dangerousness and health care costs in ways that are not applied equally to other applicants. One INS officer even informed me that, for tourists, 'it might be OK if the person takes their medication'. It is difficult to imagine similar requirements of physically ill people.

Exclusion from the US has deep historical roots. When immigration ceased to be open to all, in the late 19th century, the first groups to be excluded by law were the Chinese (thought to be undercutting white wages), paupers and the 'insane' (Chermayeff *et al.* 1991). By the early 20th century, officials at Ellis Island, New York, had about 6 seconds to detect signs of mental illness, along with certain other diseases, for example trachoma, checked by lifting up both eyelids with a buttonhook. An illustrated guide helped medical staff to identify supposed facial 'types' of mental disorder, such as schizophrenia. Doctors outlined tell-tale symp-

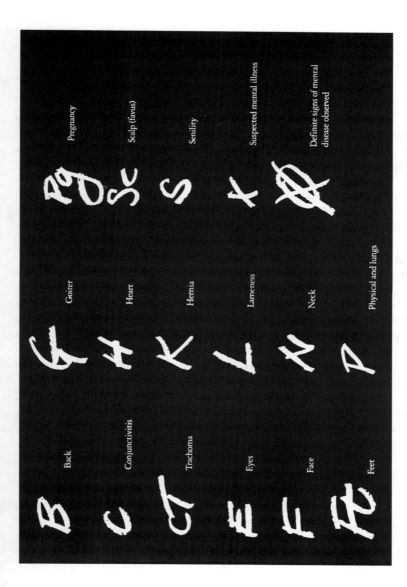

Figure 3.1 Marks chalked on the clothes of would-be immigrants by Ellis Island doctors, New York, early 20th century

toms, including 'facetiousness', 'nail-biting', 'smiling' and other 'eccentricities', as well as behaviour inappropriate to people's ethnic origin:

> If an Englishman reacts to questions in the manner of an Irishman, his lack of mental balance would be suspected... If the Italian responded to questions as the Russian Finn responds, the former would in all probability be suffering with a depressive psychosis (Dr EH Mullen, cited in Chermayeff *et al.* 1991).

If this was an early attempt to practise transculturally sensitive psychiatry, it also had severe costs for would-be immigrants. Those thought to have a mental disorder had a cross chalked on their clothing (Figure 3.1). They were then subjected to further tests for mental impairment and mental illness (Figure 3.2). Those unfortunate enough to have mental disease confirmed were duly shipped back to their port of origin, often having lost a lifetime's savings on the original ticket.

Current immigration policies descend directly from these practices. The chalk crosses have been replaced by more discreet assessment methods, but screening still prevents some people with mental health problems becoming 'Americans' or even visiting. The US is not alone in posing discouraging questions about mental illness at its borders (Campbell and Heginbotham 1991). On entry into China, foreigners are asked whether they suffer from psychosis. China and the US both have laws to prevent discrimination on grounds of disability – but these do not stop discriminatory screening at the border.

Even when people are, at least nominally, 'citizens' of the US, UK or another nation, they suffer the legacy of the beliefs, and policies, holding that people with mental illness should be segregated.

The many faces of discrimination

In 1997, a British woman, Ms X, decided to go on holiday on the advice of her GP: she had suffered an accident and become depressed as a result. Her chosen holiday company, Carefree Holidays, (she alleges) learnt of her depression, decided she would not be sociable enough for their 'carefree' holidays and turned her down.

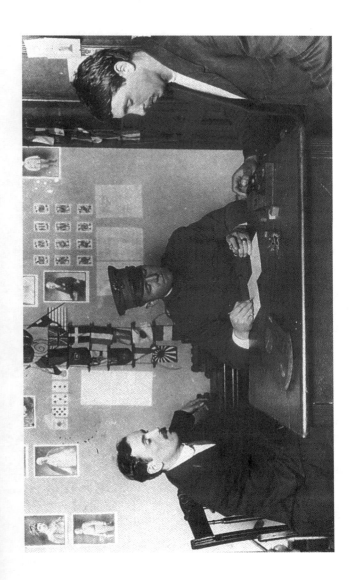

Figure 3.2   Steamship puzzle used to test immigrants at Ellis Island by Dr Howard A. Knox, circa 1916

People with a diagnosis of mental illness experience exclusion across every area of social and economic life, from holidays to work, driving cars to raising children. Discrimination may be direct, as when a mentally ill person is compulsorily medicated even when capable of giving or withholding consent, in ways that someone without mental illness could not be. It may be indirect, as for example when someone is refused a job because a 'pre-existing condition' renders him or her ineligible for an employer's health insurance scheme (Campbell and Heginbotham 1991). Discrimination may be promulgated through laws, public policies, private organisations or the acts of individuals.

Read and Baker (1996) found that, of 778 users responding to their survey: 47% had been verbally or even physically attacked (for example, having eggs thrown at them while being called a 'nutter', or dog faeces or lit paper pushed through their letter boxes); 62% said that they had been treated unfairly by family or friends and 50% by general health care services. Twenty-five per cent had been turned down by insurance or finance companies because of their psychiatric record.

The nature and intensity of discrimination varies by the diagnosis and visibility of the mental health problem (Repper and Brooker 1996) as well as by whether it is compounded by other discriminations, such as racism (Wilson and Francis 1997, Health Education Authority 1998). People with a diagnosis of schizophrenia seem subject to the most vicious assumptions, but a past history of brief depression can also lead to rejections by employers, insurance companies and the like.

Discriminatory actions are matched by cultural representations of 'otherness' that echo and reinforce unfair behaviour. A number of themes emerge repeatedly in media constructions of people with mental illness, in academic literature on the underpinnings of stigma and discrimination, and in the writings and comments of user/survivors.

The moral taint

People with mental illness are portrayed as morally lacking – shameful, dangerous, irresponsible. A stock of 'ideal types' and narratives flows through both fictional and non-fictional accounts of mental illness: the psycho-killer – usually male, often black; the pathetic, useless neglected person – often homeless; the person, often female, enabled to break through her psychological distress (for example, through the catharsis of a radio phone-in); the person whose craziness is used as a source of humour. The problem for user/survivors is that the 'psycho-killer' narrative is overwhelmingly more common than all the others put together.

Take film and TV drama. In the US, Gerbner (1990) found that 73% of prime-time TV characters with psychiatric problems are portrayed as violent. He found massively more villains for every hero among characters with mental illness than any other minority group. For every 100 physically disabled heroes, there were 12 disabled villains, and for every 100 African American heroes, 20 African American villains; but for every 100 mentally ill heroes, there were a massive 106 mentally ill villains. Programme makers may have begun to accept that it is unethical always to make black people the 'baddies', but they have no such compunction about user/survivors. Films such as *Shine*, which combine elements of the 'pathetic' and 'humorous' stereotypes of mental illness with the major theme of 'winning through' (pianist David Helfgot finds a fulfilling life, marriage and music), are a rarity.

Wahl (1995) lists a truly awesome number of both films and TV shows about mental illness in which the presence of a mentally ill villain is used to add the suspense of the unknown and to explain the bizarre. The denouement frequently involves the 'psychokiller' himself being killed, in what is presumably meant to represent poetic justice. Wahl derives the following examples from the *Washington Post* TV guide:

> *Maniac Cop 2* (1991): A monstrous former cop joins forces with a serial killer who preys on strippers in Manhattan's Times Square District.

> *Killer* (1989): A soulless maniac with a penchant for flesh slices a corpse-laden path through the Southern countryside.

> *The New Avengers*: A demented genius plots to take over the world using an army of birds.

As Wahl puts it 'there is probably no detective hero on primetime television who has not been faced with a mentally ill villain to apprehend'.

Precisely similar narratives dominate factual media coverage. It is as though we only have a few 'stories' about mental illness and slot everything – fact and fiction – into them. In Britain, Philo *et al.* (1993) found that two-thirds of the media coverage of mental illness made a link with violence. Similar findings emerge from the US (Gerbner 1990). Images of black people often predominate. In 1997, *The Times* ran an article on community care that featured photographs of five users who had committed homicides: three were black men (*The Times*, 16 July 1997). Research into homicides in fact shows that over 80% are committed by white people (Report of the Confidential Inquiry 1996); thus, a fair representation would show at most 1 black face in 5.

Homicides will always be news, but saturation exposure of the rare occurrence of homicide by user/survivors makes murder a defining feature of mental illness. The mental health lobby has not yet succeeded in firmly inserting other narratives to dislodge this particular, fear-inducing tale.

In the meantime, in order to produce something 'new', journalists invent new variations on the old theme of dangerousness. In 1995/96, a new discourse emerged in TV talk shows and magazine articles: how to protect yourself from people you know – or think you know. *Cosmopolitan* ran a feature under the headline: 'Your Man's a Major Nutcase. How Come You Didn't Notice Until Now?' It went on to advise, 'rich and adorable but he's acting like a psycho? Forget trying to reason with this lunatic... get out!' In 1997, *For Him* magazine provided a simple quiz by which to tell whether your date was a 'rabbit boiling psychotic' – for example, if she complained too much. Humour was melded with scare at the danger, under the clear message that involvement with someone 'crazy' was to be avoided at all costs (*For Him*, August 1997).

The fact that media moguls may not have discarded discrimination is suggested by the following, reported in the Boston press in 1995. During a competitive moment between Ted Turner of CNN and Rupert Murdoch, Murdoch questioned whether Turner had 'stopped taking the lithium' as a supposed dig at the quality of CNN's news coverage (*Boston Globe*, 29 Nov 1995).

These narratives are highly distressing for user/survivors:

> Every time I read about a 'paranoid killer'... I feel like someone has put a knife through my heart (Verbannic, cited in Center for Mental Health Services 1995).

It would be surprising if such articles had no effect on reactions towards user/survivors. One study found that students who had watched a movie portraying a violent person diagnosed with mental illness were subsequently more likely to express concern about people with mental illness, and less likely to find community care acceptable, than were a control group who watched a different movie (Wahl 1995). Philo *et al.* (1993) found that media imagery could, in some instances, override personal experience. Someone who has visited a relative in a psychiatric hospital for over 20 years and never seen an act of violence still 'knows' that mentally ill people are generally violent, because she or he has seen it on TV. A US study found that 87% cite TV as one of their main sources of information on mental health, compared with 51% receiving it from friends and 29% from doctors (Robert Wood Johnson Foundation 1990). In the UK, there is higher newspaper readership, but the narratives are almost identical (Philo *et al.* 1993).

Media imagery is not synonymous with public attitude, but the idea of moral taint also emerges strongly in opinion research. A review of existing (mainly American) research on public attitudes to people with 'mental disorders' concludes: 'old and young, country and city dwellers, rich and poor, men and women, bright and dull, all regard people with mental disorders as fundamentally tainted and degraded' (Farina *et al.* 1992). Mental illness clusters with drug addiction, prostitution and ex-convict status rather than cancer, diabetes and heart disease (Albrecht *et al.* 1982). Indeed, in some instances, a criminal history may be preferable to a psychiatric one:

> On two occasions I lied when I applied for jobs. On both occasions I said that my two and a half year absence from employment was due to a term spent in prison. I was accepted for the first and shortlisted for the second. Whenever I have been truthful about my psychiatric past, I have never been accepted for a job (British man aged 30, quoted in Read and Baker 1996).

If the 'psycho-killer' image is powerful, other images of moral irresponsibility also emerge from users' experiences. For example:

> My in-laws wouldn't have me in the house for 10 years after my mental illness. My wife and daughter visited them, but I was not permitted. They had the old-fashioned view that it was weakness, that I could get

a job, could pull myself out of it. I have two lives now – one in my home town, where I don't mention my life as a consumer, and one in Montgomery where I can talk about it as much as I want (user/survivor, Alabama, 1996).

The meaninglessness of users' opinions

User/survivors' views are seen as invalid by definition. In the media, this is conveyed by the chronic absence of users' voices – everyone else, from clinician to relative, seeming more 'worth listening to' – and by articles commenting on the self-evident absurdity of the 'patients running the asylums'. A rash of such stories appeared in Britain in the 1990s, criticising Patients' Councils in high-security hospitals. In reality, users were beginning to have a say on meals and visiting arrangements, but for the media, and our culture, what could be more ludicrous than 'mad' people having a say about anything?

In user/survivors' lives, the experience of not being taken seriously by service providers is commonplace (Read and Baker 1996). Standardised mortality ratios for British people with schizophrenia are two and a half times the average, partly because physical examinations are often delayed or inadequate (Sayce and Measey 1999). Other psychiatric diagnoses also affect health care:

> I went to my GP with a breast lump... [he] sent a referral letter stating 'over-anxious patient, had nervous breakdown at age 17' (20 years ago!). Consequently I was greeted by the specialist with 'well, you're a bit of a worrier, aren't you?' Every physical illness I have had for the last 20 years has first been dismissed as anxiety, depression or stress (woman cited in Read and Baker 1996).

Similarly, complaints made to criminal justice agencies are often not pursued, as a diagnosis of mental illness renders someone an 'unreliable witness' (Women Against Rape/Legal Action for Women 1995, Home Office 1998). Yet physical and sexual attacks on users are commonplace. One study in Ohio found that 47% of women in a state hospital had been raped in hospital by other patients or staff (Crossmaker, quoted in Mowbray and Benedek 1990). Others are vulnerable in family homes or on the streets: Breakey *et al.* (1992) for example, reported that 37% of homeless men and 18% of homeless women, many of whom had mental health problems, had been victims of crime. Being disbelieved removes people's power to complain; they are then effectively without protection.

Having one's views invalidated also lies at the heart of being treated compulsorily or without properly informed consent. The MacArthur treatment competence study has found that most patients hospitalised with severe mental illness have abilities similar to those of non-mentally ill people for making treatment decisions, and that those with difficulties with decision-making often show a substantial improvement following 2 weeks of treatment (Appelbaum and Grisso 1995). Yet British law permits treatment without consent for a period of months, and a lack of information and choice to make consent meaningful still persists (Cobb 1994, Faulkner 1997). This experience leads many user/survivors to state that discrimination begins inside the mental health system. Staff attitudes can reflect those of the wider culture rather than marking a break from it. Coercion can be especially distressing if perceived as deceitful, lacking concern and good faith and failing to involve the user as far as possible (Bennett *et al*. 1993, Monahan *et al*. 1995). It can erode confidence in the system altogether. A California consumer survey found that 47% of those interviewed had avoided seeking help for fear of involuntary commitment (California Department of Mental Health 1989).

Users have spoken and written eloquently on the way in which forced detention and treatment have damaged them, comparing forced medication to rape and forced detention to being criminalised:

> I went to the hospital to get treatment for what I thought was exhaustion [that is, voluntarily]. I was locked up for 9 days... My life was turned upside down. I was 26 years old. A young father. I had participated in the civil rights movement... Never had I lost my freedom for more than a few hours. This was something different. I walked to the hospital. I voluntarily submitted to examination by the physician on duty... Unbelievably a police car was summoned and... like a common criminal I was transported under arms to a locked ward. It was obvious to me that something had gone very wrong. I needed help. I sought medical assistance and had made myself a prisoner... When I lost my freedom I lost the respect of my family and loved ones (Price 1994).

The common sense of exclusion

It is part of the obvious, commonsense assumptions of life that people with significant mental health problems need to be placed at a distance. For example:

> A sad and sorry episode in the history of British social theory is drawing to a close. The policy known as care in the community, which plucked the mentally ill out of huge Victorian asylums and sent them to live, often alone, in towns and villages, is to be reversed. Instead... they will be placed in small, secure care homes... The government deserves congratulations for taking the difficult decision to admit that a whole generation of liberal social engineers was mistaken (*Daily Telegraph*, 17 January 1998).

Rumours of the end of community care were premature, but it was not the first time that journalists had sought 'closure' on the community care narrative by reaching the obvious conclusion that users should be resegregated. They should not be left to 'roam' the streets, as the media constantly put it – an animalistic image that links fear of danger to the notion that these 'other' beings should be contained in some specialist sanctuary.

For users, this 'commonsense' exclusion can generate constant rejections. For example:

> A young man... had been going tramping for some time with this club and really enjoyed it. One day he finally felt comfortable enough with his fellow trampers to state that he suffered from schizophrenia but that it was well managed. A week later his parents received a call from the tramping club to say that they would prefer that he did not attend (Peters 1997).

Although many families and friends are supportive, this cannot be assumed. The California consumer survey found that 40% never or seldom felt safe talking to family members about their problems (California Department of Mental Health 1989). Contacts are often broken and social networks reduced:

> When I went into psychiatric hospital the Minister didn't come visit me. He always visits people when they are in hospital. But he didn't visit me. It was the same with my club – they never sent a card (user/survivor, Alabama, 1996).

A Harris public opinion survey found that 19% of those surveyed said they would feel comfortable with someone with mental illness, compared to 59% with someone using a wheelchair and 47% with someone who was blind (Harris 1991). This appears to be partly linked to perceived dangerousness: Link *et al.* (1992) found that the label of previous hospitalisation is more likely to make other people want to create a high social distance if they think of mental patients as dangerous. The slogans used in campaigns to try to keep user/survivors out of neighbourhoods draw heavily on film and media stereotypes of violence, including posters of *'Silence of the Lambs'* (used in Sheffield in the 1990s).

Geographically, users often remain segregated even though no longer institutionalised:

> The concept that people in institutions had rights was revolutionary in Alabama. No one had thought of it. But many of the transitional homes are either located way out of town – where you have to go miles to get a soft drink and no one has transportation – or in the inner city where people are afraid because of the drugs and violence. It's hard to get integrated (user/survivor, Alabama, 1996).

Rented accommodation is hard to obtain. Page (1977) sent researchers, pretending to be mental patients about to be discharged, to respond to housing advertisements. Apartments were available to 'patients' from 27% of landlords and to a control group from 83%. User/survivors also often find that housing and treatment are 'bundled' (Allen 1996). If they do not want to accept the terms of being in treatment, and engaging in specified 'constructive daytime activity', they may try to get a loan to purchase property – and be turned down by banks because of patchy employment records (Housing Speak-Out, Washington DC, 1995).

> Our lives have been a trail of tears, as real as those of Native Americans who were forced to march across this country to a wasteland called their new reservations. People with psychiatric disabilities are continually offered new homes away from established communities, in a remarkably similar way (Bureau 1993).

Exclusion from education and work occurs on a massive scale (see Ch. 2). In 1996, the British Employers' Forum on Disability pointed out that Britain had 370,000 (segregated) day centre places for disabled people but only 21,000 supported employment places to help people to find and keep work (Employers' Forum on Disability 1996). An American public opinion survey found that 39% of those surveyed thought it acceptable for an employer to refuse someone a job on the grounds of past mental illness, even if they were currently functioning well (National Alliance for the Mentally Ill 1996). Employment discrimination is sometimes blatantly based on the assumption that mental illness *per se* is grounds for exclusion. In *Lussier* v. *Runyon* 1994, the Court found that the postal service had dismissed an employee with a psychiatric disability because the supervisor feared that the employee would be violent, basing this on media reports of violence committed by *other* postal employees with mental impairments (Bazelon Center for Mental Health Law 1997a). The Office of Technology Assessment found that only 4.8% of Americans with a diagnosis of schizophrenia had a degree – compared with 17% of the general population – because of both direct discrimination and a lack of support to ensure access (Office of Technology Assessment 1994).

Even mental health organisations may be reluctant to 'take the risk', as one mental health service director put it to me, of employing people with mental health problems. User/survivors have written trenchant critiques of these double standards (see Beall 1995, McNamara 1996). Sweeney (1997) writes of what happened when she told her manager that her sickness had been caused by mental ill-health:

> From that time on they treated me differently. They had taught me not to discriminate against people with mental illness, and to advocate for their rights. But I was learning that the same attitudes didn't apply to me. Fear that mental illness could affect one of them seemed to poison their feelings towards me.

User/survivors often cannot find safety from exclusion even in the agencies that are paid to serve them.

Those user/survivors who become extremely marginalised – for example homeless and/or facing major drug problems – may find that they are not accepted within homeless or drug communities and that it is hard to survive. The Metropolitan Washington Council of Governments (1995) found that people with mental health problems were often not accepted into 12-step programmes. Breakey *et al.* (1992) found that homeless shelters often did not want people with mental health problems. Homeless people generally made about $5 dollars a day from begging; many with serious mental health problems did not even make that. People with certain mental health problems can experience difficulties in understanding what other people are conveying emotionally or socially (Farina *et al.* 1992). They may also inadvertently frighten people off: for example, one man in Washington DC stood in the middle of the sidewalk waving a paper cup at people, shouting 'change' and muttering to himself incoherently. People stepped aside or crossed the road. More successful beggars adopted sophisticated techniques, men neutralising fear by operating jointly with a woman, approaching 'cap in hand' with an apologetic statement or with humour.

On the streets, people with significant mental health problems may be excluded even from any companionship or mutual help that can occur between homeless people. A California user/survivor described how he did not speak to anyone else on the street for 4 years – and nobody spoke to him.

The experience of diagnosis

Given this overwhelming, cumulative cultural and social context, it is unsurprising that people find being diagnosed mentally ill frightening. O'Donoghue (1994) has listed common responses:

Shame:	'Oh dear, I hope no one finds out'
Terror:	'Now what will happen to me?'
Isolation:	'No one will want to know me now'
Grief:	'My life is over'
Mistake:	'It must be a mistake'
Anger:	'Why me? It's not fair'

Users I have spoken with across the US and UK have repeatedly echoed these thoughts:

> When I was diagnosed I felt this is the end of my life. It was a thing to isolate me from other human beings. I felt I was not viable unless they found a cure. I didn't even think in terms of improvement – I needed a cure. I felt flawed. Defective. (man in his 40s, Texas, 1996).

These are not problems merely of individual perception which could be fixed through explanations that people are no longer (usually) institutionalised for life or that a psychiatric diagnosis need not invalidate someone's identity. For even when people challenge the notion that they are 'defective', they encounter a world that tends to treat them as 'flawed':

> People get the look of fear on their face when you say you have a mental illness (woman in her 20s, New Jersey, 1996).

The fear of rejection is such that many users 'pass' as 'normal' where they can (Brockington *et al.* 1993). A study in Staten Island found that 89% withheld information about their condition for fear of negative reactions; 25% revealed their illness only to close family members; and 7% did not even tell their close family (Wahl 1995).

> I'm black, I've spent 8 years in jail, I've got a mental illness and I'm not educated. The parts of that people can't see are nobody's business but my own (woman in her 20s, San Antonio, Texas, 1996).

Some go to great lengths to 'contain' their secret by telling only people they trust, ensuring that nothing can get back to their employer, or their family, or whomever they fear most (Faulkner and Sayce 1997). Coming out is not a one-off decision: it is a series of risks in different situations. Actual rejection, fear of rejection and the pressure of 'hiding' parts of one's experience out of terror, rather than free choice, can leave people lonely (Read and Baker 1996).

Society may have stopped incarcerating user/survivors for life, but it has not stopped excluding them. Barriers are placed in the way of ordinary activities, which for most people make up the substance of their lives and identities. At the extreme, exclusion can operate pre-birth: women are discouraged from bearing children who could go on to develop mental health problems (see below). Exclusion also extends into death: in 1997, journalist Euan McGrory of the *Northern Echo* ran a campaign to highlight the fact that psychiatric patients were being buried in unmarked graves in British hospital grounds. In some instances, people's religious beliefs were not taken into account in burial arrangements. They were denied dignity in death, as in life, in what the press aptly described as 'the final insult'.

Some people's answer to this is to socialise with other users, to set up user-run social and work opportunities. In Alabama, some users have worked to set up their own church. However, user/survivors deserve to be able to choose between user-run events and access to the mainstream.

Segregation has not ended. Rather, it has changed. The ideas that now underpin 'discrimination in the community' are in a direct line from the ideas that underpinned segregation in institutions. A local Alabama journalist described the evolution of public opinion over 25 years:

> When the court case [concerning conditions in a large mental institution] first started 25 years ago I went into the hospital and I found a 12 year old child in a strait jacket, sitting in the sun, on the dirt, with flies going in and out of her mouth. I wrote about it using the phrase 'shielded from the light': like the dead grass in the shadow of a beautiful magnolia tree, you would never have guessed from the outside how awful it was inside. The Governor, Lurleen Wallace, went through the mental retardation wards and wept. So the public got concerned about it. They still want to know people are being treated decently. But it's one thing to say we want humane treatment. It's totally different to say these people are our equals. People don't want them living in their area' (journalist, 1996).

If the values supporting segregation have not been fully overturned, other historical legacies, too, extend their influence into the present.

Worthy and unworthy lives

A strand of 20th-century history that has received much less attention than the deinstitutionalisation movement is the deliberate policy to reduce the number of disabled people through eugenics-based programmes. In the US, from 1907 onwards, people who were 'insane, idiotic, imbecile, feeble-minded or epileptic' were forcibly stopped from breeding through compulsory sterilisation programmes. Approximately 60,000 people – men and women, girls and boys – were sterilised, often without being informed of what was being done to them (Lombardo 1983). Gould documents how one woman, Doris, was told that her operation was for appendicitis. In 1980, she learnt otherwise and was now 'with fierce dignity, dejected and bitter because she had wanted a child more than anything else in her life and had finally, in her old age, learned why she had never conceived' (Gould 1985).

The long-term aim of the sterilisation programmes was to rid society of the burden of people who were 'inadequate'. Hereditary mental defects were thought to be linked to assorted social ills such as crime, prostitution and drunkenness (Lombardo 1985). A land-mark Supreme Court case in 1927 upheld the right forcibly to ster-ilise Carrie Buck, who was purportedly 'feeble-minded'. Judge Holmes, reflecting in his judgement that our 'best' citizens may be called on to give up their lives in war, said of sterilising the feeble-minded or insane:

> It would be strange if we could not call upon those who already sap the strength of the state for these lesser sacrifices... It is better for all the world, if instead of waiting to execute degenerate offspring for crime, or to let them starve for their imbecility, society can prevent those who are manifestly unfit from continuing their kind... Three generations of imbeciles are enough (Gould 1985).

A secondary aim was 'to relieve the institutions of their crowded conditions [and in order that patients] could leave the institutions, become producers and not propagate their kind' (Virginia General Hospital Board notes 1923, cited in Lombardo 1985).

Of course, sterilisation was only necessary to their release if one assumed that they should not 'propagate'. Underlying all the argu-ments was the presumption that it is socially desirable to prevent the creation of new human beings who might be mentally ill or feeble-minded. They might diminish the gene pool, they might contribute to crime and prostitution and they might be expensive.

In Britain, a Bill for the compulsory sterilisation of certain cate-gories of 'mental patient' was proposed in Parliament in 1931 by Labour MP AG Church, but was rejected. Proponents of sterilisa-tion included Winston Churchill and early birth control advocate Marie Stopes. An unknown number of forced or coerced sterilisa-tions did occur in the UK, as we know from individual testimony from women, but there was no formal mass sterilisation programme. British law still allows the subset of mentally ill women deemed 'incapacitated' to be sterilised against their will if it is thought to be 'in their best interests'.

Many European countries – Sweden, Norway, Denmark, Finland, Estonia and of course Germany – developed deliberate policies to sterilise the 'unfit'. Policy makers in Nazi Germany adapted the state of Virginia's laws with enthusiasm. About 350,000 people, categorised most commonly as feeble-minded, schizophrenic or epileptic, were sterilised in Germany in the 1930s (United States Holocaust Memorial Museum 1996).

In Germany, it was a logical next step – and one that could be introduced without too much opposition as war approached – to start the mass killing of existing disabled children and adults. This was euphemistically called the euthanasia programme. People considered 'useless eaters' and 'life unworthy of life' were gassed in ex-psychiatric hospitals, or killed by lethal injection, or shot. At least 250,000 people with mental or physical impairments were killed in these programmes from 1939 onwards in Germany and its occupied territories. Records from the era show a meticulous calculation of the savings in potatoes, margarine, quark and jam from those people who had been 'disinfected' (killed). School mathematics books posed questions including: 'The construction of a lunatic asylum costs 6 million marks. How many houses at 15,000 marks each could have been built for that amount?' The lives of people with problems such as schizophrenia and manic depression had been declared to be not worth the expense (United States Holocaust Memorial Museum 1996).

Few records or tributes exist to the individuals who were killed. The United States Holocaust Memorial Museum archive contains specific details of just one woman, Helen Lebel, a legal secretary who was gassed at Brandenburg; she was officially listed as dying in her room of 'acute schizophrenic excitement'. At a 1997 London exhibition of art produced by psychiatric in-patients in the 1920s, a number of the artists were noted to have been killed in the so-called 'euthanasia' programme (Beyond Reason 1997).

Forced sterilisation and mass killing are ethically different. It is more grave for the state to commit murder than to restrict individual autonomy in relation to invasive medical intervention and fertility, yet the philosophical underpinnings in terms of social vision are identical. Both rely on a distinction between worthy life and 'life unworthy of life'. Both justify reducing or eliminating the 'unworthy' for the sake of the economic and genetic 'good' of 'society' – assuming that one sees society as being made up only of the 'worthy' and its 'good' as keeping it that way.

One might hope and assume that this appalling history is over. In fact, we are still living in the shadow of its ideas.

The taboo on parenting

Virginia's forced sterilisation law was repealed in 1974, those of some other American states in the 1980s and Sweden's in 1976. However, just as people were to some extent freed from the view that their genes meant that they should not breed, they were confronted by the view that they could not make good enough parents. In the 1960s and 70s, laws emerged across the US that curtailed parental rights: by 1985, 23 states had laws permitting such terminations solely because the parent was 'insane', an 'idiot' or of a similar generalised category (Stefan 1989). Childbearing by people with mental health problems no longer simply spelt bad nature: it spelt bad nurture.

Despite no body of evidence suggesting that people diagnosed as mentally ill are necessarily unable to parent (Mowbray *et al.* 1995) – they can make good, bad or indifferent parents – Stefan (1989) has shown that parents diagnosed as being mentally ill lose custody for reasons 'that would rarely constitute grounds for termination with "normal" parents, such as bad attitude or sexual promiscuity'. They are also often persuaded or coerced to have abortions or use long-lasting contraception. Women may be given little recognition for the fact that they may desire the valued role of 'mother' compared with that of 'mental patient', especially since other roles, such as worker, are often not available (Sayce 1997c).

User/survivors have described separation from their children as 'a personal holocaust' (Cogan 1993), a 'grief like you can only grieve for death' (Price, personal communication, Washington DC, 1996). Sometimes they have committed suicide as a result (Perkins 1992). Sometimes they are not permitted contact with the children after adoption, despite a lack of evidence that this is in the child's interest; it may rather be in the interests of the adoptive parents. Some parents describe how the fear of losing children affects them:

> My worst fear was of losing my children. I think it actually prolonged the mental illness, because I was so scared and there was no one to help with the kids. If only there had been someone there to help (woman, Austin, Texas, 1996).

In 1996, a British survey found that, of those users responding who had children, 48% of women and 26% of men believed that their parenting abilities had been unfairly questioned (Read and Baker 1996). For example:

> My consultant psychiatrist told my husband and I not to have children –
> 'they will be taken away, no doubt about it'. We now have a beautiful two
> and a half year old daughter; we are, to quote our GP, 'excellent parents',
> and our care of our daughter is 'always of a high standard' (mother aged
> 33, quoted in Read and Baker 1996).

In the US, some cities and states have tried to address these issues systemically. In New York State, a task force was set up to look at the needs of the 10,000 children in their foster care who had at least one parent with a mental health problem, and at the needs of the parents. They began to incorporate family concerns into all policies and procedures, to develop self-help and support groups, increase supported housing for user/survivors with children, provide training for the family courts and increase information for user/survivors. However, they sound a cautionary note:

> Administrators and service providers need to be prepared to encounter
> discriminatory attitudes, particularly from the press, but also from
> some providers. At times during the task force process it was implied or
> even stated that people diagnosed with severe mental illness should not
> marry or have children because they are too fragile psychologically,
> carry a genetic predisposition, or are incapable of providing a stable
> family environment (Blanch *et al.* 1994).

In Chicago, innovative work was developed: advocating successfully in the 1980s to change Illinois state law so that parental rights terminations could no longer be based on mental illness *per se*; introducing objective standards of risk assessment; developing the Mothers' Project, which provides intensive support to parents with mental health problems and their children, including a therapeutic day programme, outreach to people's homes and help with loaning toys, securing benefits, work, housing and more (Zeitz 1995). Specialist hospital and out-patient services were put in place and the components of a comprehensive service articulated (Miller 1992).

Progress was made in Chicago until 1992, when a woman with mental health problems had her child returned to her and killed him, in a crime that became front-page news both locally and nationally. Editorials churned out the view that decision makers were obviously stupid to have allowed a woman with schizophrenia to have custody of a child – not just in this case, but (implicitly) in any case. Subsequently, custody decisions involving parents diagnosed as mentally ill became more cautious. Parents awaiting decisions stated that they felt they were being tried for the crime of the other woman who killed her child.

The media coverage did not make any reference to the fact that some women diagnosed with schizophrenia were bringing up children successfully in Chicago, with support. As a society, we have still not publicly articulated the possibility that some people with mental health problems can parent. They sometimes need support to do so (which could be funded by diverting resources from fostering and costly court cases).

There is no incentive for judges and other decision makers to take even the most carefully planned risk. If they terminate parental rights unfairly, there will be no outcry. If they make one decision in a lifetime that results in harm to a child, they will face trial by media.

In other fields, such as employment, there is now some commitment to offering disabled people support to enable them to have access to work. There is no equivalent in the field of parenting. Vocational rehabilitation tends to ignore parenting, partly because it has had a greater focus on men's than women's needs and has therefore neglected the 'work' of parenting.

In recent years, there has been a resurgence of commitment to genetic explanations of mental illness, which means that, once again, people with mental health problems are being discouraged from having children for genetic reasons – or for a combination of reasons of nature and nurture. This was the experience of Kay Jamison, professor of psychiatry at Johns Hopkins University:

> In an icy and imperious voice that I can hear to this day he [the physician] stated – as though it were God's truth, which he no doubt felt that it was – 'You shouldn't have children. You have manic-depressive illness'. I felt sick, unbelievably and utterly sick, and deeply humiliated. Determined to resist being provoked into what would, without question, be interpreted as irrational behavior, I asked him if his concerns about my having children stemmed from the fact that, because of my illness, he thought I would be an inadequate mother or simply that he thought it was best to avoid bringing another manic-depressive into the world. Ignoring or missing my sarcasm, he replied 'both'. I asked him to leave the room, put on the rest of my clothes, knocked on his office

door, told him to go to hell, and left. I walked across the street to my car, sat down, shaking, and sobbed until I was exhausted (Jamison 1995).

Many user/survivors appear to have picked up in exaggerated form the idea that any child they have will have the same mental health problems as themselves. (In fact, the great majority of children born to people with a diagnosis of schizophrenia do not develop it; 89% of those who do, have neither parent affected and 63% have no history in first or second degree relatives) (McGuffin *et al.* 1995, Darton 1998b). Even if they do develop schizophrenia, does that mean that they should not be born? As the disability community has so eloquently put it, it is not necessarily better to be dead than disabled (Golden 1991).

In 1997, the mental health charity Mind held a conference on mental health and parenting, at which a mother with a diagnosis of schizophrenia – Anne Walton – talked of how she helped her son to deal with her experiences. She entered into dialogue with the adult daughter (Karen Hardman) of another mother with mental health problems. Karen had been separated and denied any contact, letters from her mother had not been passed on (Hardman 1997). Radio and press examined the human costs for all parties in these separations. The taboo on 'mentally ill' people parenting was perhaps on the brink of being broken.

As a society, however, we have still not thrown off the idea that it is a 'mercy' to prevent people with mental health problems having and raising children. They might well taint their children, genetically and/or through bad nurture. This makes a profound, implicit statement about the worth of people with a diagnosis of mental illness. If we do not want them to reproduce, or to influence the next generation, their qualities must be fundamentally undesirable. In this sense, there has been little substantial change since the case of Carrie Buck in 1927.

Historical continuities

From a turn of the century standpoint, we are quick to spot recent changes in mental health policy and practice, such as hospital closure programmes. It is harder to notice the deep continuities of belief, and the treatment of users – although it is often apparent to users:

> We are truly an outcast people. Anti-stigma work is about re-discovering common ground. Otherwise we'll always be the 'other'. We led the parade to the death camps and no one questioned (Mary Ann Beall, Virginia, personal communication, 1996).

In 20 years' time, the continuities will be more apparent. It will be clear that, by 2000, we had changed the place and organisation of services and opened up some new opportunities, but not effectively challenged the whole notion that people with mental health problems are inferior. We have not successfully made the case to the public for full citizenship.

This raises the critical question of why the movement for deinstitutionalisation – based on ideals of dignity and individuality – did not succeed in challenging the fundamental devaluing of user/survivors that underpinned segregation.

The unfinished history of segregation

In 1950s and 60s America, black people finally won the argument that segregated education, buses, lunch counters and the like were

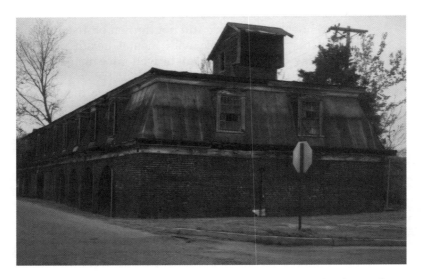

Figure 3.3   Bryce Hospital, Alabama: the building that housed black patients until de-segregation in the 1960s

not a case of 'separate but equal' (as the Supreme Court had decreed in 1896). *Brown* v. *Board of Education* (1954) determined that segregated education could not be equal, by definition.

During the same period, users of mental health services were also segregated, in institutions. In some states, black patients were housed in separate hospitals or separate wards of lower quality. For example, at Bryce Hospital in Tuscaloosa, Alabama, the basic, low brick building that housed black patients until the 1960s (Figure 3.3) can still be seen alongside the Grecian-style main building that used to house whites, with its dome, pillars and balconies (Figure 3.4).

Discrimination was held in place through forced physical segregation, in separate and unequal conditions. Patients in general were forcibly separated from the lives and citizenship rights of their original communities, and black patients were separated into places with worse conditions than those provided for whites (although conditions for white patients were also difficult). A white member of staff informed me that, in the 1960s, he had been reprimanded for associating too closely with black staff (they had sometimes travelled to work together).

One might have expected at the defining moment of black civil rights success, when 'separate but equal' was overthrown, that the justification made for segregation of people in mental institutions – providing restful asylum – would seem equally hollow. If segregating black patients within a mental hospital was now to be dismantled, what did that mean for the general segregation of both white and black psychiatric patients?

Movements for change in the mental health world of the 1960s were, however, influenced primarily by other strands of thinking. Goffman's critique of total institutions focused not on segregation *per se* but on the loss of identity and competence produced in nonpermeable, rigidly structured organisations. His analogies were with prisons, concentration camps and army camps. He did not note the resonances with wider experiences of segregation, as they applied at that time to black people and to disabled children in segregated schools – and as they apply now to users of mental health services living not only in institutions, but also in the 'community' (Goffman 1961).

Different commentators have explained the deinstitutionalisation movement that swept through the US and Europe in the postwar period in terms of new understandings of the impact of institutionalisation, hopes of financial savings, the fluctuations in

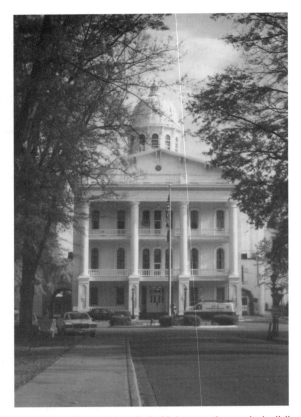

Figure 3.4   Bryce Hospital, Alabama: the main building
housing white patients until de-segregation in the 1960s

labour market trends requiring more of the marginal labour force
to be available for work, the availability of new drug treatments
or the influence of the work of therapeutic communities with
returning soldiers damaged by war (Jones 1960, Clare 1977,
Warner 1985, Pilgrim and Rogers 1993). The explicit influence of
civil rights successes, especially by and for black people, took
time to unfold.

One legacy of Goffman's work is that where community
mental health services are criticised, this is often done through
the lens of opposition to institutions – hence the derogatory terms

'institution in the community' and 'mini-institution'. These arguments, while valid in as far as they go, imply that community mental health services would be acceptable if only they would cease to resemble institutions: if they were smaller, less rigid, more permeable. This is a limited goal. It fails to set as an aim changes in the whole social environment, that would break down the barriers of exclusion from economic and social life. It fails to require that one role of mental health services should be to facilitate social inclusion.

Meanwhile other 1960s 'anti-psychiatry' writers highlighted the value of existential, rather than medical, understandings of mental illness (Laing 1960) or argued that mental illness was an erroneous concept used to defend the use of compulsion – which should be replaced by a libertarian notion of freedom of the individual to seek treatment or not as she or he wished (Szasz 1971). These critiques envisaged major changes in the way in which psychiatrists conceptualised experience and related to user/survivors, but they did not actually set an expectation that society should learn to include those with mental health problems. If anything, they assumed that once damaging institutions were removed, what was called 'mental illness' would disappear, a piece of optimism that was not born out over the next two decades (Barham and Hayward 1995).

The broader disability movement began to pursue civil rights in the 1960s with, for example, the successful campaign by Ed Roberts, who was quadriplegic, to enter the University of California at Berkeley, in the same year that James Meredith, a black student, successfully entered the University of Mississippi, escorted by US marshals (Shapiro 1993). It took time for this direct challenge to segregation to gain sway among disabled people. The first American law debarring discrimination on the grounds of 'handicap' – the Rehabilitation Act of 1973 – was not 'the end of a hard-fought battle. Disabled people did not even fight for it. Nor had they lobbied for it. Section 504 of the Rehabilitation Act of 1973 was no more than a legislative afterthought' (Shapiro 1993).

The mental health user movement, perhaps because of the overwhelming issue of the power of psychiatrists to detain and treat people compulsorily, took longer to place a priority on rights to participate in social life. There was no well-known mental health service user battling to be accepted on to a university campus. By the late 1970s, however, Judi Chamberlin had written her agenda for user-run alternatives to psychiatry (Chamberlin 1977). By the

1980s, mental health service users were working alongside disabled people to achieve the landmark civil rights law, the Americans with Disabilities Act. In addition, Chamberlin was writing of the 'civil rights movement' for mental health consumer/survivors (Chamberlin 1994). The civil rights conception broadened the base of critique, from objecting to the powers of institutions and psychiatrists, which for many users form but a small part of life, to objecting to discrimination in society as a whole. Through this lens, institutionalisation was but one form of forced segregation, objectionable because it was rooted in distinctions of value between different groups of people. And while society may reasonably segregate people in specific circumstances – such as punishment for crime, or perhaps protection from harm – the segregation of mentally ill people when others would not be segregated is experienced as an insult, a judgement that they are not worthy to mix with others (Lindow 1996). This explains why extreme segregation, like forced seclusion (solitary confinement), can be experienced as the ultimate rejection:

> When I was really hurting I was put in isolation… This experience gave me an invisible suitcase of shame that I carry with me wherever I go. The experience of being separated from other people when I was severely hurting translates into 'Don't let anyone know how bad it is or you will be left alone' (Yates 1995).

In the UK, where black civil rights successes seemed far more distant, the notion that broad civil rights were significant took still longer to surface. In 1978, the mental health charity Mind wrote to the Minister with responsibility for employment enclosing a dossier of cases of employment discrimination; he replied doubting that there was sufficient discrimination of this kind to merit new law (Bynoe *et al.* 1991).

The movement for community care has tackled total institutions, which are, in a sense, a symptom of segregation and the profound discrimination on which it rests, but it has not tackled discrimination or segregation *per se*.

Conclusion

Deinstitutionalisation and the community mental health movement have opened up real opportunities for some people, by giving them a degree more liberty, a chance for user-led organisation and consciousness raising, and the possibility of taking the initiative to pursue new avenues. For example:

> I feel very lucky. I've recovered more through this job than through years of therapy and medication – although those helped too. I really love my work – and not many 'normal' people can say that (user/survivor, Alabama, 1996).

For many people, however, life is a series of interlocking, often mutually re-inforcing, exclusions. A boy is excluded from school for behavioural problems, which makes finding work hard later – still more so after a spell in psychiatric hospital. Once he's 'flipped', his girlfriend leaves and his friends don't want to know, and there's no money, and he doesn't want the help of psychiatric services after they locked him up – and so it goes on, again and again, in many different particular patterns, similar traps, through many different lives.

When deinstitutionalisation began, it was heralded as a way of offering the chance of being in the 'community', a hope some commentators have described as a 'romance with the idea of community' (Rochefort 1988). However, although new ideas, narratives, and practices have been developed in some quarters (as we saw in Ch. 1), they have not infused our culture. It is still filled with the notion that users are blameworthy, shameworthy, to be invalidated and avoided. The values underpinning segregation, and the practices of segregation, have not been replaced.

Mental health user/survivors face barriers – located around the workplace, the neighbourhood and the friendship circle – that are rooted in the idea that socially disabled people do not have a human value equal to that of others. The continuation of the values underpinning the eugenics movement is most evident in the eagerness with which policy makers and practitioners still prevent user/survivors from parenting. Citizenship stops short of the right to bear and raise children. But these barriers permeate the culture, including through the mass media and entertainment industry. And still discrimination against mental health user/survivors goes virtually unnoticed in public debate.

At present, user/survivors enjoy only the illusion of citizenship.

CHAPTER 4

Models of Anti-discrimination Work: The Brain Disease Model

Ideals and dashed hopes

If deinstitutionalisation has not fundamentally changed the values underpinning segregation, do we have a model now that is sufficiently robust not to lead to future disillusionment? This chapter explores the contradictory aims of different 'anti-stigma' approaches and looks in detail at one of those most in favour, the brain disease model.

Some commentators believe that, so far, 'progress' in mental health policy has involved no more than going round and round in circles. Every new idea has been round at least once before: for example, the beliefs of the 1960s community mental health movement could best be described as 'archaic' (Bair 1982) as they recapitulated the humane 'moral treatment' approach of the early 19th century. Each time we have a point on the cycle at which public and policy attention is high – as in the mental hygiene movement of the 1910s and 20s and the community mental health movement of the 1960s – strong claims are made for future progress, only to be followed by backsliding and disillusionment. People with mental health problems are alternately 'discovered, forgotten and rediscovered'.

The 1980s and 90s are seen as a low point of 'decline and confusion' (Rochefort 1988), one of a number of 'periodic retreats to containment, control and avoidance of mutual responsibility' (Hudson 1993). Scull (1995) has linked recent disillusionment to the over-optimism of the 1960s, which he compares with the hopes of those building mental asylums in the 18th century: well meaning but flawed endeavours.

Cyclical models can, however, exaggerate disillusion by implying that every optimistic idea is inevitably doomed. Yet community care policies stemming from 1960s ideals have brought real improvements in numerous people's lives (see Ch. 1). Exaggerations of failure – 'like the poll tax, rail privatisation and Norman Lamont, Care in the Community is instantly associated in the public mind with failure', as the *Today* newspaper put it in 1995 – can legitimise political decisions to return to an old *status quo*: increased coercion and segregation (Sayce 1995a).

Handy (1994) argues that the proponents of change have to start building a new idea, on a 'sigmoid curve', while the last idea is still peaking. The idea of 'community care' has peaked, lost some of its power to mobilise action. It is time to build and seek some consensus on the next model.

Worlds without mental health discrimination: competing visions

According to Leighton, policy communities, during periodic retreats from ambitious reform, hit the 'Lord Ronald syndrome'. Lord Ronald was a literary figure who mounted his horse and rode madly off in all directions. When ambitious goals are not realised, groups can stop collaborating and engage in a competitive struggle for limited funds, 'thus mutually interfering with one another while dissipating the resources' (cited in Rochefort 1988).

In any era, different stakeholders – user/survivors, family and friends, providers, policy makers and corporate interests – hold visions of the future informed by different and sometimes conflicting interests. In the current climate of relatively low morale, collaboration and shared agendas may be especially scarce.

Different groups invest considerable energy in tackling the problem of discrimination. They do so on the basis of widely varying, often contradictory, conceptions of what a world without discrimination on mental health grounds would mean. While there is near-universal consensus on the need to dislodge the old idea of the sin and shame of mental illness, there is almost no agreement on what should replace it. Even if the aims were clear, there is still relatively little evaluative evidence on which methods of reducing 'stigma' or discrimination work (see Chapters 8–12), so people can also 'run madly in all directions' in their choice of methods.

Key players tend to believe that improved public understanding would reduce discrimination, but their ideas vary on a number of axes, for example:

- what the phenomenon of 'mental health problems' is: a number of discrete diseases (schizophrenia, manic depression and so on), or rather points on an unbroken continuum from health to ill-health, or a set of labels that exist only in the eye of the beholder.

- what causes the phenomenon: genes, faulty neurotransmitters, early object relations, a loss of spiritual harmony, social disadvantage or oppressive diagnostic labelling.

- what should be done to reduce discrimination: explain that mental illness is a biological disease like any other; or argue that no one is 'mentally ill' – if we abandoned medicalising diagnosis then stigma, caused by labels, would fall away; or promote universal emotional openness and thus show that, far from no one being ill/distressed, we all are – all being on the same continuum; or revalue being different and seek access and inclusion for user/survivors as a distinct minority.

While these beliefs are not all mutually exclusive – many people believing that genes and social disadvantage combine to cause mental health problems, or that diagnoses are socially constructed and also describe real differences in feeling and behaviour – they tend to cluster in ways that produce highly contradictory accounts of how discrimination is best tackled. For example, promoting the idea that mental distress/illness is something we all experience is in direct contradiction to arguing that mental illness is a disease just like cancer – which many people never experience.

Others have produced categorisations of the different understandings of the nature and causes of 'mental ill-health' (see especially Pilgrim and Rogers 1993). Here, I identify four common conceptual models used specifically in the quest to reduce stigma or discrimination. There are overlaps and variations on these themes, but most practical examples of anti-discrimination work fall within one or other of these frameworks.

The brain disease model

'Open Your Minds: Mental Illnesses are Brain Diseases'. Thus ran the headline for the National Alliance for the Mentally Ill's (NAMI's) 1996 anti-stigma campaign. On this view, the hope of the future rests with science. As the genetic and biochemical roots of problems such as schizophrenia and severe depression are gradually uncovered, the public will come to see that a disease of the brain is no different from a disease of any other bodily organ.

At the core of this view is the notion that a brain disease is 'no fault': it is not a moral weakness, not the fault of the parents, not caused by the environment. It can instead be understood at the level of physiology. It is morally neutral, and by removing blame – from any party – we shall take the sting out of the discrimination currently faced by service users and their families.

A 1993 video on the history of NAMI describes two defining moments in the growth since the 1970s of this movement led by family members. The first was coining the term 'brain disease'; the second a challenge by a family member to the notion of parental blame:

> I was in Massachusetts and a woman said to a group of professionals, how many of you here believe that families cause mental illness? Quite a few hands went up. She looked at them and she was shaking all over, because she'd never been making any public performance before. And she said, 'then don't have anything to do with families, because they can see it in your eyes'.

The video ends with a father of someone with mental health problems stating:

> I tell my wife it's a brain disease. It's nobody's fault. You're a good woman.

One critic of the 'brain disease' approach told me that, in her view, family members had, very understandably, 'jumped for the first explanation that did not blame them'. Barney (1994) notes that this is because of the absence of discussion in the mental health community of the well-documented impact of the wider, socio-political environment on people's mental state. For example, Rodgers found higher rates of mental disorder in adults who had lived in council housing in childhood and who had been in care;

multiple childhood disadvantages compounded the effects (Rodgers 1990). Albee, reviewing epidemiological studies, found that 'the very poor are at highest risk for many pathological conditions, including mental disorders'. He also reported that those in the US with the highest rates of mental disorders were currently landless migrant farm workers; historically, as successive waves of immigrants moved out of poverty, the rates in those communities declined (Albee and Ryan 1998). Perkins and Silver (1994) found that unemployed people in a London borough were eight times more likely to be referred for mental health problems than those who were employed. The design of these studies indicates that poverty and disadvantage are not only the consequences of being diagnosed mentally ill: they can also be causative (Albee 1992). While these understandings remain relatively hidden, families are left with a choice between two explanations: 'a defective family or a defective brain. Not surprisingly, the latter is usually chosen' (Barney 1994).

If, in 20 years' time, the no-fault brain disease conception has prevailed, its advocates would predict a number of benefits. People with brain diseases will no longer face discrimination in access to treatment: as a medical condition, brain disease will be covered in all insurance policies, not merely on the basis of full parity *with* treatment for physical illness but *as* a physical illness. It is, perhaps, only a matter of time before policy makers recognise that the brain is a physical organ like any other.

This conceptualisation will revolutionise how society and the law attribute responsibility. As the schizophrenia gene or genes are mapped, and the underlying biochemical imbalances more fully understood, the 1960s Laingian notion that family upbringing contributes to what is called mental illness will finally be consigned to the dustbin of history.

We shall see that people with brain diseases are not responsible for their illness – and equally not responsible for actions, such as crimes, that they commit when ill. As Fuller Torrey put it, 'violent acts are usually part and parcel of the illness' (Fuller Torrey *et al.* 1990). They are usually preventable through treatment. We shall therefore look back with disbelief at the 1990s figures for people with mental illness residing in jails. A 1992 survey by NAMI and the Public Citizens' Research Group found that, in many areas, people with mental health problems were in jail for minor misdemeanours such as drunkenness or trespassing; once there, they were cruelly abused by other inmates (Fuller Torrey *et al.* 1992).

By the 2020s, there will have been a massive expansion of forensic psychiatry services, as tens of thousands of prisoners are transferred into secure hospitals for treatment. The name of Varnall
Weeks, a man diagnosed with paranoid schizophrenia who was
executed in 1995 in Alabama, will be cited as a prime example of
the barbarity of a distant era. Mr Weeks believed that he was God
in various forms and that upon his death he would reappear as a
tortoise in the sky (Southern Center for Human Rights 1995). As far
as the Court was concerned, this meant that he had sufficient
understanding that he would die and could therefore be executed.

Finally, a hugely increased number of people will seek help as
the stigma of blame is removed. In many cases, effective treatment
will prevent suicide and wasted lives.

For critics of the 'brain disease' model, this dream has all the
qualities of a nightmare. It has been criticised, first, by organisations concerned to protect the interests of people with mental
health difficulties that are not or are not proven to be 'brain
diseases', for example children with severe emotional disorders. If
non-discrimination in public policy depends on a person having a
physical brain disease, that relegates other mental health problems
to the second tier – to no health insurance coverage (in the US) or a
low priority for the NHS (in the UK), and little public understanding. As Rubenstein put it in an open letter in 1996, the NAMI
campaign 'perpetuates as well as fights discrimination'.

Some states in the US have passed laws providing parity
between physical illnesses and biological brain diseases – but not
mental illnesses in general. At a federal level, this was only averted
in the mid-1990s by counter-lobbying, by the Bazelon Center and
others, against proponents of insurance parity for 'brain diseases'.

By 2020, the balance of power between lobbying groups might
have shifted, and we might see a greater neglect of people with
problems stemming from long-term exclusion, or war, abuse and
other trauma, as well as the abandonment of people who did not
choose to identify with the concept of brain disease. They might
come under considerable pressure to replace psychotherapeutic,
or social, or spiritual, understandings with biological ones – or to
face the loss of mental health services, social security, anti-
discrimination protections and so on. The explanations that help
some people to make sense of their experiences – their childhood
or rootlessness or state of grace – might be eclipsed in the interests of privileging biology. Susko (1991) argues that the psychiatric system already 'treats any spiritual phenomenon as a

symptom of a neuro-chemical imbalance'. This could become more pronounced.

As genetic testing develops, we could all – for a few dollars or pounds a test – be divided into those with 'pluperfect' and 'imperfect' genes, as the US Congress put it, and genetic discrimination could be set to grow (Gostin 1993). We shall know our genetic make-up as we now know our blood group. If tests were to be successfully developed for a predisposition to manic depression or schizophrenia, those with mental health problems could be divided into people with 'real' brain diseases and those with no brain disease. We might see a growth of support groups for people in specific genetic categories, including those with no genetic justification for their mental health problems, who might face a new 'stigma' – being seen as malingerers. Meanwhile, those with 'real' brain diseases might face different discriminations: for example, being discouraged from bearing children in order to protect the gene pool from the lethal mix of genes for mental disorder and violence, and to safeguard the economy. In Britain, the law already allows for abortion up until full term in the case of a disabled fetus but otherwise puts the limit at 24 weeks, a situation that has reasonably been described as a eugenics-based law (Kennedy 1996). Those with serious impairments born when they could have been aborted or genetically engineered might encounter discrimination on every front – no healthcare, and blame attached to them and their parents for not bowing to the demands of science.

Ethicists working on the human genome project may prevent some of these imagined excesses. However, this scenario does suggest that the concept of 'brain disease' is not automatically benign in its potential impact on discrimination. Other critics have fundamentally challenged the notion of 'brain disease' as inaccurate and dangerous.

It is seen as misleading because it tends to overstate biological causation. A correlation between changes in brain chemistry and changes in feeling and thinking does not mean that the first caused the second. It may equally be the other way round, or a third factor may cause both: severe emotional trauma may lead to psychological problems and to changes in neural pathways; or neuroleptic drugs may cause changes in the brain that then get picked up on brain scans and interpreted as evidence of the 'abnormalities' of schizophrenia (Breggin 1991). NAMI campaign materials nonetheless list 'accurate' public perceptions of the cause of these disorders as genetics and biochemistry, and 'inaccurate' perceptions as family and environmental factors.

This is not supported by the available evidence. Take genetic causation. While debate rages about the existence of the schizophrenia gene or genes, studies suggest that much of the variance in the development of schizophrenia is not explained by genetics (see Ch. 3). Geneticists and ethicists themselves often stress that the study of genetic predisposition should go hand in hand with the investigation of environmental factors, and that high heritability does not mean that environmental interventions are 'a waste of time' (Parens 1996, Rutter and Plomin 1997).

Yet proponents of the 'no-fault brain disease' tend to assume no significant environmental causal effects. This is taking moral neutrality too far. It leaves little room to discuss toxic forces in people's environments that have a known potential to damage mental health: relative poverty (Gunnell et al. 1995, Gomm 1996, Wilkinson 1996, Henderson et al. 1998), poor housing (Huxley et al. 1989), unemployment (Jahoda 1979, Warner 1985) and, in some cases, although it is understandably taboo in family movements, abuse or neglect within families (Brown and Harris 1978, Mullen et al. 1988, Palmer et al. 1992, Herman 1994). Reducing all mental health problems to biology masks the environmental forces that ethically, as a society, we may decide to address. In this sense, mental health problems are not entirely 'no fault'. They are biological, in the sense that every thought and feeling is a physiological event, but they need to be understood through a lens that scans a person's interactions with his or her whole environment – and which is prepared to make ethical judgements, to spur action to tackle poverty, gender discrimination and other patterns of inequality that impact on people's mental health.

Given continuing increases in income differential, social divisions and concern about crime (see Ch. 2), genetic explanations could become increasingly useful to justify this particular *status quo*. Murray and Hernstein (1996) argued, in *The Bell Curve*, that the 'underclass' is anchored at the bottom of American society by its unfortunate biology and that social programmes for the 'genetically inferior' are therefore a waste of money. In 1995, Glayde Whitney, outgoing President of the Behavior Genetics Association, asserted that 'it is a reasonable scientific hypothesis that some, perhaps much, of the race difference in violence is caused by genetics'; by implication, it is therefore justifiable that American jails are so disproportionately filled with black men. Critics note that these arguments are 'correlational garbage': they mistake associations between genetic difference and behavioural difference for cause and effect. They might be dismissed were it not for the fact that *The Bell Curve* hit the best-seller list and that cuts in social programmes such as Headstart appeared in part to be justified by the argument that African American children were less bright than white or Asian children, and therefore unlikely to achieve, whatever support systems were in place (Favre 1995).

In this climate of opinion, the 'failures' of people with mental health problems can readily be attributed to faulty genes rather than to the way in which social exclusion often keeps people in a vicious circle of poverty, mental health problems and worsening poverty.

In public and media debate, there is a huge conflation between mental illness, violence and being black (as we saw in the previous chapter). Genetic arguments can be used to explain the violence in society by recourse to the genes of black people and mentally ill people – and especially black mentally ill people. The most obvious solutions engendered by this set of understandings are genetic engineering, selective abortion, and medication to mitigate the effects of genetic disorder – ideas that raise the spectre of attempts to reduce the number of black mentally ill and other disabled people in society, as opposed to ensuring that they are valued and accommodated in workplaces and other communities (Asch 1989, Pfeiffer 1994, Favre 1995). And if aberrations in behaviour are increasingly interpreted as mental illness – 'do mental health professionals think anyone is normal?' as Caplan put it (see Ch. 5) – a powerful mix of behavioural genetics and the genetics of mental illness could be used to explain, or over-explain, a variety of behaviours that society wants to see reduced, from sexual nonconformity to rude behaviour in schools.

As long ago as 1970, Levine and Levine argued that explanations of mental disorder in terms of the individual's internal make-up would flourish in socially conservative times, as they 'assume the goodness of the environment' (Levine and Levine 1970). More situational approaches, which question the social environment, flourish during periods of political or social reform, when the *status quo* is anyway being challenged. Or as Lombardo put it in 1995, 'Convenient, isn't it, that in a time of serious budget cutting, suddenly scientific theories advocate taking money away from the poor and powerless?' (quoted in Favre 1995). In this sense, purely genetic explanations let society off the hook.

One simple test of effective anti-discrimination work must be that it does not compound discrimination. Overstating genetics fails that test: it occludes the way in which discrimination affects mental health, thereby reducing the scope of anti-discrimination strategies; it privileges more biologically caused mental health problems over others in a discriminatory way; and it compounds fixed and prejudiced views of people in the so-called 'underclass', especially black people, and black mentally ill people. Geneticist Gottesman admits that, in the current climate, a whisper of genetic influence tends to be turned to a shout of total genetic control. Mental health advocates need to help to tone down the shouting.

This does not mean denying all genetic influence on mental health problems, as some user/survivors and allies have done in order to deflect discrimination (Breggin 1991). That also fails the anti-discrimination test. Rather, this approach assumes that people who do have a proven genetic predisposition to impairment can be discriminated against with impunity. It also runs counter to basic science, which suggests that environmental and genetic influences are inseparably interwoven from conception onwards. The mental health movement needs to challenge genetic discrimination – for example, to rectify the absence in UK disability discrimination law of coverage for people facing discrimination on the grounds of genetic predisposition. A genuinely anti-discrimination position is one which says that people with mental health problems should not face discrimination, irrespective of the causes and not one that implies, 'don't reject us – we're not like the others, we have a genetic problem which we can't help', or conversely 'don't reject us, we aren't part of the genetically inferior underclass, we have just been damaged by circumstance'.

The 'brain disease' model appears naïve in assuming that stressing genetics will of itself make discrimination wither. While, at first glance, genetic explanations may seem to offer some protection from moral censure, the history of forced sterilisation and the eugenics movement shows that saying one was 'born this way' is no automatic protection. History gives little comfort to those who believe that if only the public knew that mentally ill people 'could not help it', they would readily come to respect and value them.

The notion that discrimination can be overcome simply by emphasising genetic causation falls precisely into the category of wildly over-optimistic approaches cited by the cyclical analysts: such approaches fail because they oversimplify. They do not address the huge number of interlocking facts at stake.

If the 'no-fault brain disease' position is problematic in assuming 'no responsibility' on the part of politicians or the wider society, it also removes responsibility from user/survivors in ways that can damage their chances of full citizenship. The idea can have some appeal for user/survivors, especially as a counterblast to older views of madness as some form of divine retribution:

> I always thought it was something I'd done. The biological approach to mental illness does help (woman user/survivor, Texas, 1996).

For others, understanding in terms of lived experience, rather than just biology, has the same effect. However, the 'no-fault' brain disease model also argues that people are not responsible for their actions (see Fuller Torrey 1990, and above), which leads straight to patronising attitudes and a denial of rights:

> People used to be called crazy and lunatic. A lot of hatred was directed at them. NAMI stepped in and said no, don't hate them, they're sick. Pity them. Now we're stuck with a lot of pity. I wish someone had had more foresight and substituted something different for the hatred (woman user/survivor, Massachusetts, 1995).

The denial of user/survivors' capacity to take responsibility is based on a presumption of a lack of judgement, which provides the philosophical basis for involuntary commitment and forced treatment. This is considered by many users to be the worst discrimination of all (see Ch. 3). The laws and policies permitting compulsory treatment – which for other citizens would be considered assault – in fairly broad circumstances, stem not from hatred but from a paternalistic notion that users cannot take decisions in their own interests. It is therefore only fair – and compassionate – that someone else take decisions on their behalf, with the pre-eminent aim of restoring them to health. If user/survivors try to point out that, for some, avoiding forcible injection is more important than a reduction of symptoms, they are seen as 'lacking insight'. This leaves them no way whatsoever of asserting their own priorities where these differ from those of professionals.

Mental health problems do not obliterate judgement. They can make thinking so difficult that society may decide it should intervene to ensure safety – often for very short time periods (Grisso and Appelbaum 1995), and often in ways that can be resolved through advance planning when the person is well, through advocacy or simple creative thinking: for example, problem solving with someone within their own frame of reference, rather than resorting to force.

The corollary is that people with mental health problems tend to have responsibility if they commit crimes: their whole judgement is not nullified just because they have a diagnosis of, for example, schizophrenia. There may well be mitigating factors: their social circumstances, contingent on the exclusion they experience as user/survivors, and sometimes particular aspects of their mental health problem – such as extreme mood swings, leading them to drink excessive alcohol – which makes the crime more likely but does not make it inevitable.

Society has some significant responsibilities towards user/survivors, for instance to prevent discrimination (see Ch. 2), but this does not mean that user/survivors have none. Removing responsibility from people is to deny their humanity. It leads to the most paternalistic and abusive tendencies of welfare provision. It is possible to interweave social and individual responsibilities in such a way as to depart both from old-style welfare paternalism and from individualistic models of consumer choice, which so easily ignore the power imbalances that make 'choice' a chimera.

A non-discriminatory position is one which recognises that mental disorder *per se* does not invalidate judgement. Many citizens make unwise decisions. User/survivors should not be expected to be any wiser than anyone else. Overruling someone's decision – even when it seems, to well-motivated professionals, to be an unwise decision – must be heavily constrained. And if users commit crimes, it should not be assumed that it is not their fault.

The 'no-fault' position has in practice, as well as in theory, underpinned efforts to increase compulsory treatment. Critics note that NAMI has recommended more compulsory treatment in jails (Fuller Torrey *et al.* 1992) and in the community (Albee and Ryan 1998). When Senator Kassebaum introduced a bill in 1995 to make homelessness funding to states dependent on their having outpatient commitment laws – that is, laws permitting involuntary treatment outside hospitals – NAMI was a lone voice in favour. The measure was defeated by user/survivors bombarding Senate offices through the Internet and by lobbying by the Bazelon Center for Mental Health Law.

NAMI as an organisation does not base all its work on a pure 'brain disease' model. It has campaigned vigorously for employment rights and opportunities, and does not assume that people with 'brain diseases' are consistently incapable.

These splits along the fault line of views on forced treatment are repeated in Britain. SANE, like NAMI, emphasises a genetic, 'no-fault' position, and was one of only two organisations that supported the Mental Health (Patients in the Community) Act 1995, which brought in greater controls over user/survivors, including provision allowing for police to 'take and convey' people to day centres against their will (Sayce 1995a).

Some critics of the 'no-fault' position – for example, Washington-based activist Ron Thompson – have argued that the emphasis on biology in the 'brain disease' model is in itself the basis for forced treatment. This is an oversimplification. Those with a clearly organic brain disease such as Alzheimer's disease should have the right to make decisions for themselves on all the issues on which they are able to make choices safely – and the right not to be under-estimated or overruled.

There is one final critique of the 'brain disease' model: that it privileges medical treatment over other approaches such as psychotherapy or self-help (Breggin 1991). This does not follow as night does day. Many people receive therapy for organic brain disease (Sacks 1985) or antidepressants when their marriage breaks down. However, there are strong marketing forces at play that aim to reinforce the link between biological problems and biological solutions. They use the resonant cultural image of the scientist uncovering biological causes, identifying scientific cure, in order, directly or indirectly, to sell products.

Pharmaceutical companies have increasingly used awareness raising with the general public as a marketing strategy – instead of directing marketing efforts only at prescribers (witness, for example, the high public profile in the 1990s of the antidepressant Prozac). The 1996 NAMI campaign, cited above, was largely funded from the marketing budget of a pharmaceutical company, Eli Lilly. This company has a global strategy of increasing the proportion of health budgets spent on drugs. It has purchased information tech-nology companies that can provide information to physicians on health care options for specific diseases. It thus aims to provide 'healthcare solutions that will often be both clinically and economi-cally superior to alternative forms of treatment – in effect, the ther-apeutic substitution of pharmaceutical-based solutions for other forms of treatment and intervention', to quote its Chairman, Randall L Tobias, in his 1995 address to shareholders. During the

1990s Eli Lilly opened offices in sites ranging from Kazakhstan to Cairo, Argentina to Beijing; by 1996, it was selling products in 150 countries. By 1995, world-wide sales of Prozac alone exceeded $2 billion, and 21 million people had taken the drug. Sales of all their products rose from $3 billion in 1987 to over $6 billion in 1996.

In order to 'open up' or extend markets, Eli Lilly works with at least 150 groups – like NAMI – to promote messages that fit with their marketing strategy: for example, that depression can be effectively treated in 80% of cases, that brain diseases should have parity with physical illness in health insurance and that spiritual understandings are not sufficient for serious mental illness. Eli Lilly has supported the American Association of Pastoral Counsellors, which has produced video and other teaching materials for religious leaders, encouraging them to recognise mental illnesses and refer people to doctors – as they would for physical illnesses: in effect, to complement pastoral counselling with medical help. While these materials were produced in a Judaeo-Christian tradition, they make reference to mosques and are being used internationally across differences of culture and religion. The video gives a balanced depiction of the role of different causal factors in mental illness. It also mentions the importance of pastoral counsellors verifying that the illness has a biological component, which can give a 'kind of pastoral permission to do something medical' about it (American Association of Pastoral Counsellors 1995).

Some religious outreach, for example that run by NAMI, has included significant efforts to ensure that religious organisations genuinely include user/survivors, offer them work and make them fully part of congregations. Pharmaceutical marketing, too, can have beneficial effects in user/survivors' terms, for example, reducing the shame associated with mental illness by raising its profile publicly. But while companies – of which Eli Lilly is just one example – are pursuing legitimate business interests, these do not precisely match the interests of user/survivors, but they are, of course, far better funded than user-run initiatives are ever likely to be.

A particular 'mismatch' occurs on the issue of compliance: pharmaceutical companies have a vested interest in improving 'compliance', whereas user/survivors reject the entire concept, having even convinced the Royal Pharmaceutical Society in Britain to abandon the term, with all its implications of obeying someone in authority. They chose the term 'concordance' instead, on the grounds that it gives a greater sense of a partnership between user and prescriber (Royal Pharmaceutical Society of Great Britain 1997).

Pharmaceutical companies are major players in anti-stigma work. They fund defeat depression campaigns around the world – which generate vast numbers of articles, from *Readers' Digest* to women's magazines, stating that depression is treatable. The 'chance to see' that single message about treatability must run into thousands of millions. These companies favour the 'brain disease' notion: it can more easily be linked to the promise of heroic scientific breakthrough and cure than can more 'messy' environmental, social or spiritual understandings (as evidenced by the slides of magnetic resonance imaging (MRI) brain scans that typically accompany media work on these campaigns); it underpins the strategic goal of substituting the prescription of medication for other therapies.

User/survivors do not universally want to adopt biological understandings, nor pharmaceutical solutions. Some do; many find drugs helpful. But in terms of messages to the public, many would prioritise the idea that user/survivors should be valued whether they get 'cured' or not. The 'treatability' message is of little use to those who remain depressed. In addition, many would want more coverage for other possible remedies, such as social support or therapy (Rogers *et al*. 1993, Faulkner 1997). The 'free market' in this instance provides wide opportunities for messages that suit some vested interests but far less exposure for others.

While anti-stigma campaigns based on these models have rarely been evaluated, where they have the results have not necessarily been beneficial from user/survivors' perspectives. A Norwegian study found that an anti-stigma campaign succeeded in making people more likely to recommend that someone in distress seek help from a doctor or other professional and correspondingly less likely to recommend talking to friends or family about their problem (Fonnebo and Sogaard 1995). This might be deemed a 'success' in relation to the objectives of a pharmaceutical company, but for user/survivors, feeling less able to talk to friends and family could actually exacerbate the painful impact of discrimination.

It is not the case that the brain disease model inevitably leads to medication-based solutions, but, given the level of resources being channelled into making that link by pharmaceutical companies, it is indeed a likely outcome. Anti-stigma efforts using the 'brain disease' model are currently prominent in the US and to a lesser extent in the UK. Some campaigns have taken a less hard line than NAMI's, but the link to medication is still strong. For example, the National Mental Health Association's

1993 educational video 'Moving into the Light' includes a doctor explaining that mental illness is not a weakness but is caused by a number of factors including genetics and chemical imbalances. Although other influences on mental illness are mentioned, they receive less prominence. The remedy most strongly advocated is psychiatric drugs.

By funding non-profit organisations, companies are enabled to convey their message, or a variant of it, through an organisation that appears to have no vested financial interest, thus potentially vastly increasing the message's credibility. The difficulty for non-profit organisations is how to promote different messages, that give the public a wider range of insights into discrimination and the position of user/survivors in society, on anything like the same scale.

Conclusion

The 'no-fault' brain disease model removes the moral taint of mental illness but raises new difficulties on numerous fronts. Allocating no fault, and no responsibility, is fundamentally problematic in terms of the sharing of rights and responsibilities necessary to citizenship. Additionally, the power of the vested interests pursuing this model means other messages, especially those promoted by user/survivors themselves, are easily eclipsed.

The question is, has anyone created more promising models for combating discrimination? The next 3 chapters examine the other significant models that have been employed to reduce discrimination – beginning with approaches aiming for individual growth.

CHAPTER 5

The Individual Growth Model

This model tears down distinct disease categories, or at least minimises their importance, in favour of a single line, stretching from 'emotional well-being' at one end – including the capacity to learn, achieve autonomy, be self-aware, enjoy relationships and meet challenges – to ill-health at the other. We are all somewhere on this line. We move up and down it. This 'continuum' notion has underpinned much mental health promotion work. It is influential in the traditions of counselling and psychotherapy (Pilgrim and Rogers 1993) and New Age spirituality (Coward 1989) as well as in users' critiques of the damage inflicted by psychiatric labels (see, for example, Wallcraft 1996, Foner 1997).

In this model we shall, in 20 years' time, stop seeing 'mental illness' as a minority problem faced by other people. Therapy will have become like glasses, as one activist put it to me – something that used to be rare but lost its stigma as most who could afford to engaged in it. This will destigmatise mental health problems because we shall recognise that we all have some distress or pathology to tackle, we can all reach higher levels of awareness – and no one should face discrimination for having the courage to embark on their own personal journey.

The benefits of this model are seen as increased emotional and/or spiritual literacy for the population at large, analogous to improved vision, and an abandonment of the narrow, rationalistic, 'macho' suppression of emotion in favour of a new openness of heart and/or spirit (see, for example, Goleman 1996). It offers user/survivors the prospect of understanding experience through a variety of frameworks – early childhood influences, spiritual dynamics – which may accord more meaning than a straight biological approach, which tends to ignore the content of people's thoughts and feelings except as an indicator of pathology. At best, the idea of the continuum could be used to emphasise the common humanity of everyone with or without diagnosed 'mental health problems'.

The pure 'therapy as glasses' version of this view is somewhat on the defensive in the US, and more recently the UK, for reasons of economics. During the debate on Clinton's proposals for health care reform in 1993/94, a huge lobbying effort by the Bazelon Center and others succeeded in getting mental health care included in planned coverage – against considerable opposition from insurance companies. This was achieved by accepting strict limits for psychotherapy, which, advocates conceded, was not necessarily cost-effective, but gaining more elastic limits for medication (Koyanagi 1995). Parity would never have been accepted if opponents could have argued that this would fund Woody Allen-style psychoanalytic indulgence. Rationing requires categories – and resists models based on a continuum approach that could generate limitless demand. In the event, the whole health care reform fell, but achieving parity in principle paved the way for efforts at state level and for more limited federal legislation, passed in 1996, that specifically mandated parity between mental and physical health care in private insurance. The price for getting mental health covered at all was a general reduction in the status of psychotherapy.

In Britain, a series of Department of Health reports on the effectiveness of psychotherapy has emphasised the cost benefits of short-term focused counselling and therapy, especially cognitive therapy, and noted that therapy can be cost-*in*effective when it lasts too long (NHS Executive 1996). Locally, this has been translated into increases in short-term focused counselling/therapy, with less attention to longer-term, especially psychodynamic, approaches.

Put bluntly, in a climate promising public funding constraints for the foreseeable future, it is improbable that therapy will become a long-term aid – like glasses – for anyone bar the professional and moneyed classes. In Britain, right-wing think tanks and the tabloid press have tried hard to ensure that it does not. The Social Affairs Unit's paper *Magic in the Surgery* argued that 1 in 21 of the workforce was engaged in providing 'counselling' (a figure which it arrived at somewhat bizarrely by including all police officers and social security officials); that this 'state licensed friendship service' was eroding traditional morality by insisting that anything was 'right' if people 'felt comfortable' with it; and that since it was unscientific, ineffective or downright damaging, it should not be provided on the NHS (Harris M 1994). Tabloid newspapers went on to publish sensational stories of therapists threatening the moral order of society and family by 'implanting' 'false memories' of abuse in their clients (see Kitzinger 1996, Sayce 1996).

By the mid-1990s, psychotherapy was on the run, its advocates thrown on to the defensive. They appeared unable to compete, in their public and marketing messages, with the biologically framed ideas that were hitting doctors and the general public about the treatability of mental illnesses/brain diseases, nor with the banks of research data apparently demonstrating the superior cost-effectiveness of drugs. Some cut their losses by joining forces with advocates of biological models, in campaigns advocating counselling as an appendage to medication.

But we do not all have to partake in therapy to be influenced by its ideas. Psychoanalytically derived thinking still permeates our culture (even if its decline may have begun). Many people have built concepts such as subconscious feelings and defence mechanisms into their world view. There are also other channels for 'individual growth' than psychotherapy: the ever-popular alternative/complementary therapies, which treat not brain diseases but a person's whole physical, emotional and spiritual world; 'lifestyle' health promotion activities, which aim to enhance positive mental health rather than only treat or prevent illness; and spiritual and growth movements.

Access to some of these approaches is also likely to be limited. Despite a considerable demand from users for therapies ranging from acupuncture and herbs to massage (Faulkner 1997), such forms of help are primarily available in the for-profit sector and are not normally covered by private insurance. Also, many 'growth movements' are at least as expensive as psychotherapy, as the opulence of the lifestyle of their gurus attests. The alternative health movement has begun to take steps to accumulate effectiveness data (see, for example, Wallcraft 1999) but not to the extent that it shows any immediate sign of competing successfully with other corporate interests for an increased share of mainstream health resources.

Growth movements and New Age and spiritual approaches come in many models, but all share a belief that everyone is capable of 'growth'. Several of the movements most actively involved in promoting public messages on mental health place themselves in direct competition, ideologically, to biomedical understandings.

Re-evaluation co-counselling, which promotes specific ideas on mental health through literature and conference presentations, understands 'distress' (rather than illness) as a response to being hurt and oppressed. 'Mental health system survivors are people who are neither "crazy" nor "mentally ill" nor genetically distinguishable from anyone else' (Re-evaluation Counseling Communities 1991). It sees no role *at all* for psychiatric drugs, advocating instead that people counsel, cry and laugh to 'discharge' their distress. One proposal is:

> To expose and eliminate the deep hurtfulness of 'mental health' system 'treatments'; in particular, the loss of life, diminished capacities, imposition of terror and grief, and prohibition of joy and excitement from such 'treatments' as psychosurgery, electric convulsive 'therapy', drug 'therapy', isolation, and incarceration. These 'treatments' must stop.

It accepts 'no limits to human functioning': 'All people can eventually, with the complete elimination of their distresses, function well in every respect.'

The Church of Scientology, which claims eight million members world wide, has published a series of booklets on the various ways in which psychiatry is said to have betrayed women, black people and others. It shows a video to people interested in joining, which states that psychiatrists and psychologists are criminals. Since the growth of the community mental health centre movement has coincided with rises in crime, drug use, illiteracy and other social ills, these problems – scientologists argue – have been directly caused by the infiltration of psychiatry and psychology into schools, courts and society at large. This is perhaps one of the most grandiose attempts ever made to use a set of correlations to assert a causal link (Citizens' Commission on Human Rights 1995). Scientologists propose a solution called 'audit', which is claimed to succeed where psychiatry and psychology fail (although when I asked about evidence, the answer was that one has to experience scientology by joining in order to understand). Unsurprisingly, scientologists have come into direct conflict, including in the courtroom, with pharmaceutical companies promoting their products.

Do individual growth movements reduce discrimination?

Even if access to 'individual growth' remains constrained, the cultural values of emotional literacy, coupled with the combined effects of all the personal growth activities, might in principle reduce discriminatory attitudes and/or behaviour among those members of the public who partake in them. The evidence for this is not especially promising.

Most evaluations focus on whether or not the approach 'heals' rather than on its impact on discrimination. There is some evidence that the presence of counselling in American and British culture through TV counselling programmes has enabled viewers better to clarify their own problems – although not necessarily to alter their behaviour (Barker *et al.* 1993) – and, for participants, to reduce the stigma attached to seeking help (Burns 1997). Perhaps this is partly because our cultures so value 'fifteen minutes of fame' that exposure on TV adds to a personal sense of status rather than reducing it. Oprah Winfrey and her successors may keep alive the idea that we can all benefit from talking about our problems, although whether modelling 'talking' to millions of invisible viewers from cultures as diverse as China and Mexico actually adds to people's ability to talk privately, to friends and family, may be open to question. Burns (1997) also notes that TV exposure can harm a minority of those participating and Larson that the sensationalism of the programmes can be exploitative (Larson 1981, cited in Burns 1977). The women who choose to confront on camera, for example, their sisters for having affairs with their husbands may create dramatic television, but they leave hanging a question of some sadness – of whether anyone in their personal circle has witnessed their experience or offered support.

The fields of mental health promotion and illness prevention may be based on a single continuum (health to ill-health) or two linked continua (health to ill-health, cross-cut by positive to negative well-being, such that one person could have no ill-health but equally no positive well-being) (Downie *et al.* 1990). Programmes using both models have demonstrated some successes in terms of enabling people to move towards health and/or positive well-being. Programmes have improved coping skills and self-esteem in *general* populations, for example schoolchildren (Tilford *et al.* 1997, Durlak 1998), and in *at-risk* populations. For instance, Pedro-Carroll and Cowan (1985) found that support for children after divorce led to significant improvements in assertiveness and anxiety levels. Clarke *et al.* (1995) found that groups for adolescents at risk of depression reduced the number of students with mood disorders by 56% in 17 months and Gillham *et al.* (1995) found similar results in relation to at-risk 10–13-year-olds. Durlak (1998), reviewing 177 studies of primary prevention with children and young people, found positive mean effects in every category of intervention bar one; effectiveness was maintained over time. Achievements have been documented in relation to both strengthening the capacities of groups (for example, by enhancing support networks) and changing environments. For example, Felner *et al.* (1993) found that multiple changes in a school environment reduced depression, delinquent behaviour and school drop-out. Albee and Ryan (1998) noted that individual 'lifestyle' approaches, encouraging individuals to change their behaviour, are insufficient when the environment is toxic. There is also no specific evidence that any of the 'positive mental health' or preventive interventions reduces discriminatory attitudes or behaviour faced by people with mental health problems; rather, they may, in some cases, reduce the risk of people developing mental health problems in the first place (National Institute of Mental Health 1994, Tilford *et al.* 1997).

The co-counselling movement runs workshops on mental health oppression, which appear to raise the awareness of discrimination among participants. Otherwise, while debate rages about the effectiveness, or lack of it, of alternative therapies and growth movements, there is no specific evidence for their impact on discrimination.

Critiques of the individual growth model

Many writers have commented critically on therapies and growth movements generally, in terms of the power imbalance built into the very nature of the therapeutic relationship (Masson 1988), or indeed into the relationship between movement leaders and their followers (Bunting 1996). Also discussed have been the culture of blame created by alternative health and growth movements, as personal 'responsibility' for health shades inexorably into blame or self-blame when someone develops cancer or depression (Coward 1989), and the potential of therapies to weaken the ability of intelligent communities to solve their own problems, by bringing in outside 'experts'. Other authors have investigated the diversion of energies from collective responses to political problems, into individual self-reflection (Wilden 1972, Kitzinger and Perkins 1993) and the 'marginal' potential impact of individual therapy given the structural nature of people's difficulties (Pilgrim 1997). Numerous other commentators have criticised one model in order to boost another.

In the context of the claim for growth movements and therapies that they offer 'meaning' rather than biological reductionism, it is worth noting that each tends to do so in its own, often somewhat prescriptive, terms. For many user/survivors, if they have any 'choice', it is between one view being foisted upon them and used to interpret their world and frame their solutions – or another view. There is a competition between groups with different world views, intensified by constrained budgets and fuelled by the groups' interests in enhancing the status of their profession, the resources for their service, the size of their movement or the bottom line for their product. While users' views have in theory to be listened to, services do not respond quickly to users' priorities: Faulkner (1997) found an almost identical set of complaints about an over-emphasis on drugs at the expense of listening, as had been found by Rogers *et al.*, whose research was conducted over five years earlier, a period during which users articulated their demands repeatedly and consistently (Rogers *et al.* 1993). People diagnosed as mentally ill simply do not have power as 'customers'.

My emphasis, here, however, is on whether the 'individual growth' model has the potential to reduce discrimination on mental health grounds. In this respect there are a number of problems.

First, the notion of a 'continuum' may in some ways entrench the very idea of a polarity between the positive associations of health and the intractable negatives of ill-health that the model is supposed to disrupt. If one finds oneself at the 'lack of health' end of the line, it is unclear why one would derive value simply from being 'on the same continuum' as everyone else, any more than the pupil with the lowest marks in a class that values high marks would feel reassured by being 'in the class'. Groups who use the continuum idea in an attempt to get rid of the negative notion of mental illness find themselves thrown into euphemism in describing the negative end of the spectrum: 'lack of health' and 'ill-health' side-step the term 'mental illness', but only just. By emphasising the positive, the ability to aspire to 'higher' points on the continuum, there is a risk of devaluing the lives of people who do not move 'up'. Downie *et al.*'s (1990) double continuum goes some way to reducing this problem, as one can have both a 'mental illness' and positive well-being, but it has not been widely adopted in mental health promotion (Secker 1998).

The 'individual growth' model is fundamentally about providing prevention, healing, cure and self-improvement. Many people want cure. Many people who cannot have 'cure' want improved health –

in the sense of a greater fulfilment in life. But we also need a mental health equivalent of the argument adopted by people using wheel-chairs: 'I do not accept imagery, and heroic stories, that suggest my life is worth living only if I "walk again"; I want to be accepted as I am.' It is in the interests of providers of every sort of therapy and spiritual growth to offer solutions – of varying hues – for people seeking healing, and to use the continuum theory to point out that huge numbers, even all of us, can benefit. This should not, however, be confused with a movement or a set of messages that fundamentally offer respect and social inclusion to people who hear voices, or believe they are being persecuted, or are depressed.

Although mental health professionals have often chronically underestimated the potential of people with mental health problems to recover and lead fulfilling lives (consider, for example, 'every professional gave up on me, including the anti-shrink shrink': Unzicker 1994), the opposite tendency can be equally oppressive: the person who 'discharges' their distress, or undergoes 'audit', and still does not 'function' in every sphere of life, as was claimed, can take on a terrible sense of failure. In addition, it is difficult to imagine a doctrine further removed from 'mad and proud' (see Ch. 1) than the 12-step commitment to being 'restored to sanity' by admitting one's moral shortcomings to a 'higher power': the implication is that one should be ashamed until the mental illness has gone.

It would be possible to ditch the health–ill-health continuum and opt for a simple scatter of different specific experiences, some common, some rarer, for example hearing voices, or feeling extremely anxious, or having to check and double-check on every task completed. This places no positive or negative value on these experiences: voices can be inspirational or punitive; obsessional checking can be useful for someone whose job is to check pharmacy prescriptions but debilitating for someone who never dares leave the house. The scatter model does not risk implying that some people's lives are somehow less valuable, because less healthy, than others, but it can address the discrimination faced because of unusual experiences. It gives scope for including multiple concepts of 'health', whereas single definitions tend inevitably to the culturally specific (as in the white, Western, male notion that the key characteristic of health is individual autonomy or mastery) (Secker 1998). It also addresses a further problem with the continuum: that a single 'line' is probably not credible with the public, not a concept that 'works'.

An early piece of Canadian research evaluated a public education programme based on the 'continuum' model (Cumming and Cumming 1957). The authors tested attitudes before and after a six-month educational campaign designed to promote more accepting attitudes towards people with mental health problems. The community – a small town – rejected the entire programme, as they could not accept that normal and abnormal behaviour fell within a single continuum. While it could be argued that this reflects a common fear of being associated with, on the same continuum as, 'mad' people – which might be rectified by further educational campaigns – it is equally likely that people simply find it hard to obliterate the differences between, for example, thinking you are Jesus Christ, feeling sad after a relationship breakdown and being 'stressed' at work. It is indeed difficult to see in what sense these very different experiences are on a 'continuum'; they are qualitatively, not just quantitatively, distinct. Many in the user/survivor movement have been breaking down broad categories such as 'schizophrenia', whose validity is in doubt (Bentall 1990), and replacing them with far more specific experiences such as 'hearing voices' (Baker 1995), or 'self-harm' as distinct from attempted suicide (Bristol Crisis Service for Women 1994, Pembroke 1995). Far from wanting to blur all the current diagnostic categories into one notion of 'distress' or 'continuum', users want to get past diagnosis to a greater level of detail. As that happens, the differences between hearing voices and stress at work, and between hearing different kinds of voices, become ever more marked, and the continuum notion is stretched to breaking point.

Some spiritual and religious work on mental health also draws very fine distinctions. Maitland (1997) has noted that Saint Theresa of Avila, in the 15th century, distinguished between visions that came from God, those from the devil and those caused by madness. One could tell the difference by asking whether they brought joy and added to the well-being of the whole community, in which case they were Godly and must be shared, whether they produced unhappiness, egotism, selfishness and destruction, in which case they were devilish, or whether they were incomprehensible, in which case they were mad.

As we search to find languages that reflect the breadth and depth of the experiences of madness and distress – languages that fit different cultural and spiritual frameworks – we are horribly limited by the notion that there is one 'continuum'.

There is also a strong likelihood that use of the 'continuum' notion in education campaigns destigmatises more minor problems at the expense of people who are more disabled. One of the model's proponents said to me, 'We need to put forward images that people can identify with – and if we say mental illness is schizophrenia, that scares them off'. A number of educational videos focus only on people who appear totally 'normal': for example, the National Mental Health Association video 'Into the Light' is introduced by someone who is not overtly a user but is famous (the actor Rod Steiger). Once he has reassuringly and 'normally' framed the issues, a number of user/survivors are interviewed, none of whom gives any evidence of significant difference from the norm in their thinking or feeling.

Some advocacy organisations reinforce discrimination by avoiding giving air-time to the very people who face the worst discrimination, for example young black men with a diagnosis of schizophrenia, whose only media exposure is then the photographs linking them to violent crime. One 1990s conference on challenging stereotypes included a video of user/survivors' views, rather than a live talk, because of anxiety among the organisers: at a previous conference, a user had been unwell and disruptive. Judging a class of people on the basis of one person's previous behaviour seems to typify stereotyping, which is unfortunate in a conference designed to challenge it. The message often conveyed is that user/survivors should be accepted because they are just like everybody else. This appears to leave those who are not 'just the same' entirely abandoned.

Media counselling and phone-in programmes have concentrated almost entirely on problems such as bereavement and anxiety, and rarely on problems like 'schizophrenia'. It may be no coincidence that, in a decade that has lifted the taboo on discussing these explicable problems, media constructions of 'madness' and 'schizophrenia' have become ever more demonising (see Ch. 3). We truly seem to have destigmatised one 'end' of the so-called continuum at the expense of the other.

It is only videos made by user/survivors that show people who do appear different – who shuffle from the adverse effects of drugs, or have difficulty communicating, or say things that seem odd. On mainstream TV, these user/survivors are shown only as images of pity in newsclips about homelessness; they do not speak. But in user-made videos, like the Californian 'People Say I'm Crazy', viewers are able to hear what people who do appear different have to say. This has a major potential to reduce discriminatory attitudes.

Showing only people who are 'normal acting' may destigmatise problems such as less severe depression, but where is the evidence for the 'trickle-down' theory, the idea that this will help those who are hearing persecutory voices and talking to themselves? It could instead mirror the early community mental health centre movement: placing attention on those with less severe difficulties on the assumption that this will somehow help those who are most disabled. It took years to establish that this faith had been misplaced (Mollica 1983, Sayce *et al.* 1991); we could side-step a similar lengthy process by going straight for the evaluation of a range of messages designed to challenge discrimination against all groups of user/survivors.

A further problem with the individual growth model is that it sets up a particularly risky battle about what is or is not pathological. On a continuum, potentially all behaviour – or none – is pathological. The strongest push is to pathologise more and more of life. In the late 1990s, articles in the British press repeatedly announced the 'discovery' of new illnesses: hair pulling, homesickness and shopping addiction to name but three. Research cited by the American Psychiatric Association states that just under half of American adults aged 15–54 have a mental illness in their lifetime, 1 in 5 being affected every year. This clearly provides considerable justification for the services of psychologists, therapists and counsellors – as well as psychiatrists. The American DSM (*Diagnostic and Statistical Manual*) increased the number of mental disorders from 297 in the 1980s to 374 in the 1990s. Adding pre-menstrual disorder made half a million more women pathological at a stroke (Caplan 1995). Caplan argues that this eclipses issues in the women's lives such as domestic violence in favour of neutral sounding 'syndromes'. Saying that children have 'oppositional defiance disorder', another DSM category, is perhaps rather like the old diagnosis of 'drapetomania' that was applied to slaves in the early 19th century if they ran away. Being defiant can become a disorder as the practice of diagnosis veers into the absurd.

Caplan uses these points to question the whole project of diagnosis on the grounds that it is not scientific: decisions about whether homosexuality was a disorder, for example, were made by vote. However, there is another danger, which is to campaign for the removal of particular conditions from the DSM because, for example, women who have been abused will be stigmatised by diagnosis – and therapeutic understandings show that this is not an 'illness'. The more fundamental campaign might be to remove the sting of discrimination and shame from any diagnosis, or any other system of categories – not to take out post-traumatic stress disorder but leave unchanged the low value accorded to people diagnosed with schizophrenia.

The DSM is open to considerable question as a reliable and acceptable categorisation system, but we do need a language, a set of categories, to describe different experiences. The most promising are those rooted in user/survivors' own articulations of their experiences.

The risk with the 'individual growth' model is that attempts to oppose discrimination will be fought out at the margins, over the concerns of certain groups to avoid stigma by absenting them-selves from the DSM. It will not be fought at the fundamental boundary of the difference in power, and value, and respect, and opportunity, between people who have a mental health problem (of any kind) and those who do not.

A further critical problem is that most of the approaches grouped under the individual growth model focus on individual and famil-ial solutions rather than environmental ones. A review of mental health promotion research conducted by the English Health Educa-tion Authority in 1997 found 'a critical gap in the absence of evidence on programmes concerned with the social and economic determinants of mental health. There is a strong need to support more research in areas like housing, inequality and discrimination' (Tilford et al. 1997). Work by Albee has advocated community-based change as a necessary part of primary prevention for two decades, a thesis backed by numerous epidemiological studies showing that 'poverty, powerlessness, exploitation and discrimina-tion are major causative factors' in mental ill-health (Albee and Ryan 1998; and see above) and by evidence that prevention requires both strengthening the host and reducing the toxicity of the envi-ronment (Benzeval et al. 1997, Albee and Ryan 1998). Numerous commentators, however, have noted that this emphasis on inequal-ity and poverty has been overshadowed by the scores of articles on how individuals can improve their own self-esteem and coping skills in advance of confronting stressful situations, while the situ-ations themselves remain unchallenged (Albee 1986, National Insti-tute of Mental Health 1994, Davison et al. 1997) .

A 'growing society' might be effective in reducing discrimina-tion, as well as distress, if it were self-reflexive not in terms of how people can better adapt and 'grow' as individuals, but in terms of learning collectively, from groups facing discrimination, from people living on the margins, about how patterns of inequality need to change (see Ch. 1). This is not generally what individual growth proponents have in mind.

A further area of contention is that movements such as 12-step and Scientology place 'growth' in very specific moral frameworks. For example, the 12 steps for Emotions Anonymous – for people with problems of panic, anxiety, depression, abnormal fear, self-pity, resentment, remorse, jealousy, envy, boredom and many more – include confession and living a 'better' emotional life. Getting 'better' in the sense of recovering seems to have become entirely synonymous with being 'better', that is, more moral. This holds out the horribly deceptive hope that emotional problems, contingent on real forces from sexual assault to unemployment, could be dissipated by overcoming emotions such as envy – becoming calm and at ease – rather than being spurred by envy or anger into action. This harmonious ideal may leave little space for the person who is at odds with the social environment.

'GROW', a 12-step programme designed specifically for people with mental health problems, states that people become mentally ill through 'personal failure – that is, through learned habits of false thinking and disorganised living'. One of its directors stated in 1995 that wanting to pursue political, rather than personal, change on mental health issues 'could be a way to escape changing oneself. GROW is therefore not politically active' (cited in European Newsletter of Users and Ex-users of Psychiatry 1995).

Similarly, Louise Hay's classic *You Can Heal Your Life* gives possible causes for 'insanity' – 'fleeing the family, escapism' – and suggests individual changes in thinking to bring 'healing'. Anxiety, for example, can be healed by loving and approving of yourself (Hay 1996).

These suggestions that people bring 'madness' on themselves and can think their way out of it carry an immense risk of victim blaming. Coward (1989) argues that the whole alternative health world is one 'where individual intentions, strength of will and commitment to a lifestyle which is right and harmonious have their rewards in visible good health. And it is a world where wrong attitudes – neglect of self-expression and needs – have their punishments. It is a world of heroes and villains.' She acknowledges the potential value of 'taking responsibility' in terms of escaping from passivity and personal powerlessness, but sees this particular form of responsibility as so individualistic as to present no challenge whatever to patterns of inequality; instead, it helps people to adapt, and sometimes succeed, within them. Additionally, personal transformation is constrained by the models themselves: the alternative health movements offer the chance to change into what you 'really' are. Thus does 'growth' co-exist with fatalistic philosophies such as astrology, which limits what one can be according to the position of the planets at one's birth.

Individual growth approaches, just like the brain disease model, fit Levine and Levine's notion of leaving the *status quo* unchallenged (see Ch. 4). Some models of therapy do explicitly address political issues such as sexism and racism, but they rarely actively support collective consciousness and action to redress them. Self-help books typically advocate adapting to existing conditions rather than trying to change them. *Men Are From Mars, Women Are From Venus*, for example, suggests that a woman should seek support from a man with a 'non-demanding attitude' – that is, should not diverge too much from traditional expectations of women – otherwise the man will be resentful (Gray 1992).

Discrimination against people deemed 'mad' or 'mentally ill' is a longstanding historical phenomenon. It has to be tackled socially, politically, in public debate, rather than only through an atomistic approach in which numerous separate individuals improve their own mental health.

The culture of 'personal growth' also privileges emotion over reason. Some critics argue that this anti-enlightenment, anti-intellectual trend could erode the basis for thinking strategically about how to achieve social change. For example, in Britain, some feminist and other commentators heralded the huge public reaction to the death of Princess Diana in 1997 as a sign of emotional renewal, a shift from the deathly 'stiff upper lip' culture to a new expression of moral and spiritual values. Others saw it as the triumph of sentimentality over any hope of political transformation. Wheatcroft (1998) saw a fulfilment of WH Auden's warning of a future age in which 'reason will be replaced by revelation... Justice will be replaced by Pity as the cardinal human virtue.' As Wheatcroft put it: 'the canonisation of St Diana painfully illustrates the decline of feminism – of rational political feminism, that is. Did Mary Woolstonecraft and Emily Pankhurst live for this... The rights of women they [now] vindicate are the rights to suffer, to feel bitter, and to make trouble. Diana was the perfect example of a woman who never did anything.'

While an anti-emotional culture can stifle people's lives and mental health, any movement for justice needs analysis as well as passion. It needs to resist 'settling' for cultural change that permits open emotion or commitment to every possible spiritual sect, if these are not accompanied by political and social change. If users still cannot travel, work or raise children, permission to cry is cold comfort. A New York social worker told me that she asks homeless people with mental health problems their star sign and talks astrology to them, and in the drop-in they can read the large sign that says 'In every difficulty lies an opportunity'. However, advocacy efforts to protect people from periodic police 'clean-ups' were on the decline. Growth movement philosophy links neatly to the American dream: everyone can seize an opportunity if they really try, or if fate or the stars decree it. But for most homeless people the American dream is a distant, often mocking, fantasy.

Combined brain disease and counselling campaigns

Many anti-stigma efforts in the US and UK – for example the American DART campaign to raise awareness of depression, and Britain's Defeat Depression campaign – combine the brain disease model with some degree of emphasis on counselling.

These campaigns represent alliances – between providers of talking treatments, physical treatments, drug manufacturers – based on the shared interest in breaking down 'stigma' as it inhibits help-seeking. For example, the Ohio company SERCO set up a five-state 'Fight the Stigma' campaign. They concluded from their pilot that it was possible for mental health providers to improve their market position and that 'predictions for growth in the mental health professions are positive' (Nelson and Barbaro 1985).

In 1996, a private psychiatric hospital corporation (Charter) advertised heavily on American TV, encouraging people to seek their services for severe depression. The powerful advertisement ended with the phrase 'Even if you don't go to Charter, seek help somewhere'. Companies can bargain on the idea that promoting help-seeking generally will increase the size of the overall cake. Other campaigns, such as the pure 'brain disease' approaches, may be more geared to establishing the size of their particular slice.

Conclusion

Where the biological brain disease model brings the welcome relief of removing responsibility for the 'illness' – and the terrible drawback of removing responsibility for everything else too – the 'individual growth' model gives people back responsibility for their actions. Scientology, for example, despises psychiatry for absolving rapists from blame. However, this approach also gives back responsibility for health itself, and thus implicitly blames people when they do not get better.

User/survivors might find that arguing for talking treatments or alternative therapies, rather than only drugs, is of limited help in terms of changing the overall conditions of life: increasing the options may give a heightened sense of control for some user/survivors, but there is a limit to personal 'growth' when people are constrained by real external forces such as discrimination in employment. The 'continuum' model on which much of this work is based has serious drawbacks in terms of its credibility with the public and its potential to reduce discrimination against those who are most marginalised.

All campaigns on the 'individual growth' model have as a strong focus encouraging people to seek help – which they may be prevented from doing through 'stigma'. In this respect they are very similar to the 'brain disease' campaigns, except that the type of help on offer is different and the resources available for marketing far smaller.

Encouraging help-seeking may be a valid aim, but it is also limited. Once people have sought help, they are still likely to be denied citizenship rights. In order to examine models for anti-discrimination that are more far reaching, and that address responsibility and rights in more sophisticated ways, we need to turn to those developed by user/survivors and by disabled people more generally. This will be the focus of the next 2 chapters.

CHAPTER 6

The Libertarian Model

The libertarian model is perhaps best summed up by a button (a 'badge' in UK terms) on sale at the 1995 conference of the National Association of Rights Protection and Advocacy (NARPA), which read 'Equal civil rights and equal criminal responsibility for mental patients'. It was next to buttons reading 'You bet I'm non-compliant and inappropriate' and 'Go manage your own case and get off mine'.

In this model, the core aim is to throw off the oppression of laws allowing forced psychiatric treatment. Most activists also want no involuntary commitment, which 'punishes us for what we think and for someone's fuzzy predictions of what we might do in the future, RATHER THAN WHAT WE ACTUALLY DO like other adult citizens' (Williams X 1995). Indeed, if one were to suggest incarcerating young men known to drink heavily (incidentally, a group with a worse record of violent offences than users of mental health services; Mullen *et al.* 1998, Steadman *et al.* 1998) when they were thought to be 'at risk' of getting drunk and attacking their wives and girlfriends, the civil rights implications would immediately attract comment.

Other activists suggest that if involuntary commitment has any place, it should be on the basis of actual, recent examples of violence and should be carried out explicitly because society wants to control someone – rather than being accorded the euphemistic label 'treatment'. In this way, the public will not be allowed to think that involuntary hospitalisation and treatment are some benign kind of 'help': they are examples of government overriding human rights in a way that it cannot do, in almost all circumstances, in relation to people with physical illnesses.

In this view, forced treatment lies at the very heart of the oppression of people with mental health problems – it is the 'branding iron' (David Oakes, personal communication 1996), the equivalent of slavery. To Americans, forced treatment shows that user/

survivors are not full citizens of the Union: they lack the rights to liberty and privacy enshrined in the Constitution. Outside America, users may be less attuned to thinking in terms of civil rights, but they still see forced treatment as premised on the non-verifiable notion that a user is 'unable to judge his or her own best interest' (Chamberlin 1977). Users' humanity is denied as their every decision and wish can be overridden on the spurious, and highly subjective, basis that they 'lack insight' – for example, if they disagree with their psychiatrist, whose own 'insight', given relative power positions, is not open to such scrutiny (Chamberlin 1994).

Some proponents of this model believe that diagnosis is part of the system of oppression: the whole notion of 'mental illness' is suspect, constructed in order to legitimate control through psychiatry and the law. This view was more current in the 1960s and 70s, with the writings of Szasz and Laing, than today, but it has had something of a resurgence in the 1990s through post-modernism, which throws all categories from race to mental illness into question.

Some believe that the growing influence of the 'faulty brain' model legitimates increased coercion – for example, the extension of compulsory treatment to community settings – because 'chemical imbalances' imply that judgement is, objectively, damaged. It should, however, be noted that psycho-analytic theory can also be used to undermine users' opinions (as therapists may claim understanding of a client's 'unconscious' motivations and refuse to take his or her views at face value) (see Chs 4 and 5).

Given this spectrum of views, for many members of user/survivor movements – especially in the US but also in Europe – the abolition of forced treatment is the single highest priority for campaigning. People have to get rid of this appalling government oppression before they can even consider other goals. In 1995, NARPA formalised its long-standing position to oppose all forced treatment. The European Network of (Ex-)Users and Survivors of Psychiatry also took a decision to oppose all compulsory treatment.

Campaigners have documented the damage of compulsory treatment. User/survivor literature compares forced injection and physical restraint (sometimes in the four-point position, with legs and arms outstretched) to rape, and forced ECT to torture (Grobe 1995, Shimrat 1997; see also Ch. 3). For many people who have been abused earlier in life, this amounts to revictimisation (Blaska 1995).

If, on this view, any treatment without consent is ever justified, it should be provided for legally on criteria that apply equally whether or not someone has a mental disorder. 'Mental disorder' itself should never be, as it is in British law, one of the criteria. This argument essentially defines mental health laws as discriminatory *per se*: they allow the state to coerce people with 'mental disorder' in ways in which it cannot with other citizens (Campbell and Heginbotham 1991, Harrison 1998). Rather, one might have laws that tightly define 'incapacity', for example as meaning being 'comatose or otherwise unable to communicate, and I specifically exclude people who are clearly communicating what others may not want to hear' (Chamberlin 1994). In all other circumstances, treatment without consent would be defined as assault. That way, someone actively trying to refuse ECT would never be given it, but someone who was unable to speak because of severe depression could be (assuming that ECT were still available, itself under debate; see, for example, Read and Reynolds 1996). Where possible, 'incapacity' would be planned for, so that people gave or withheld consent in advance: people would make 'advance directives' and/or nominate someone whom they would trust to act as an advocate for them.

In order to get these rights, people have to take responsibility. They cannot maintain their 'secret unwillingness to be held at least in part accountable for some of their actions while mentally ill', as activist Ron Thompson put it (in a letter to J Dart 1994). Therefore the insanity defence should be abolished. Far from wanting to divert people from jail into (implicitly involuntary) hospitalisation, as NAMI advocates, in this view people should be in jail if they have committed crimes, and if they are locked in a 'hospital' against their will, this should be a separate, clearly coercive system, distinct from any system that might also exist to 'help' people. A psychiatrist cannot reasonably be involved in both incarcerating someone and 'helping' them.

On equal criminal responsibility, Williams states: 'sure, this may mean that the handful of people who escape execution by NGRI (not guilty by reason of insanity) will die [that is, through execution], but what about the many many more who die in restraints and seclusion rooms, or of iatrogenically induced drug effects?' (Williams X 1995). Some user/survivor activists with whom I spoke in the US thought that people diagnosed as mentally ill who committed crimes – especially high-profile crimes such as the attempt on ex-President Reagan's life – were letting survivors down. They damaged everyone else's reputation and should definitely take responsibility for their actions.

A minority position holds that 'reasonable accommodations' under the Americans with Disabilities Act (ADA) 1990 are a way of not taking full responsibility at work. If employers and the public see user/survivors as people who cannot work exactly as others because their judgement is impaired, or their emotions troublesome, the corollary will be a continued belief in forced treatment. In order to be treated as full citizens, user/survivors have to behave fully responsibly. Thompson has therefore argued that the physical disability movement should distance itself from people making 'vague and bottomless claims... for mental disability in the name of reasonable accommodation'. Forced treatment and reasonable accommodation, he argues, stem from the same philosophical base. Therefore, the ADA should not be supported in relation to people with mental health problems; indeed 'justified criticism' of the ADA in relation to psychiatric disability could taint or undermine the gains made for physically disabled people (Thompson, letter to J Dart 1994).

Anti-forced treatment campaigns are not heavily funded but have achieved some successes through use of Internet lobbying, media relations and public demonstrations. Internet lobbying defeated Kassebaum's out-patient commitment proposals (see Ch. 4). In Madison, Wisconsin, a demonstration opposing forced ECT, led by survivors and a nurse challenging being fired for refusing to administer ECT without patient consent, made front-page news in the Wisconsin press and placed pressure on local psychiatric providers.

In the 1990s, Ron Thompson lobbied in Washington *against* parity in health insurance between physical and mental health care; in his view, more money for mental health could mean 'the lifelong coercion of an ever-expanding sea of mental patients' (letter to J Dart, 1994). Other Washington mental health organisations did not support him, although some grassroots groups shared his concerns. In 1997, he argued against 'women leaders for mental health' – a global initiative to reduce stigma, led by Mrs Roslyn Carter – on the grounds that 'the virtues of Mom, Apple Pie... and Volunteerism have been enlisted... [to give] every human on the planet the right to voluntary *and involuntary* mental health care' (Thompson, unpublished paper 1997).

In Britain, the pure libertarian position is less prominent than in the US, given Britain's stronger traditions of welfarism, which have placed the state as a beneficent executor of collective responsibility (through 'our' NHS) as well as an oppressor. In addition, the British user movement has objected more fiercely to the medicalisation of distress than to power itself. Thus, in 1998, when the government announced that 'non-compliance with agreed treatment will not be an option', users chose to demonstrate not against government but against the Royal College of Psychiatrists' anti-stigma campaign, on the grounds that the diagnoses of psychiatry were (they believed) the origin of 'stigma'. This anti-diagnosis, anti-medical treatment position, common in British radical user politics, limits the basis for coalitions to prevent attacks on civil rights, as it tends to exclude the many users who choose to take drugs, and the numerous psychiatrists who object to the restriction of their role to social control. Nonetheless, campaigns against compulsory treatment have occasionally been in evidence, from the Campaign Against Psychiatric Oppression of the 1970s, to campaigns against compulsory ECT, by ECT Anonymous and Mind, in the 1990s (Cobb 1993, 1994). Even these, however, tended more to the 'anti-ECT' than the 'anti-compulsion' position, as evidenced, for example, by the fact that Mind opposed compulsory ECT but not compulsory treatment *per se*.

The American survivor argument for full rights and full responsibilities is intellectually consistent and more compelling than some British liberal positions, which argue for increased rights – for example no compulsory treatment in the community – yet shy away from full responsibility, continuing to advocate for wide-scale diversion from custody.

If the libertarian position – which effectively simply asks that governments withdraw their oppressive laws and practices – prevails, we may expect that, in 20 years' time, forced treatment will indeed be perceived as analogous to slavery in the US, and be either abolished or be in the throes of a major abolition campaign across much of the world.

Critics are concerned on several fronts. First, many people want mental health services, for all their imperfections. The idea that the only anti-discrimination priority is to 'get the state off your back' can leave people fearing no support at all, or feeling guilty for wanting that support. For example:

> Some survivors can manage without medication and services. I'm happy for them. But they assume everyone else should be like them. Those of us with long-term disabilities and who need treatment – we need a voice too. When I hear that the only thing that matters is involuntary treatment I think what matters to me is people dying on the streets (user/survivor, Virginia, 1996).

The pure libertarian position is that it is not viable to argue simultaneously for the basic political right of no forced treatment and for resources from the same mental health system. Others disagree. Many user/survivors have set up consumer-run drop-in centres, accepting money from mental health departments. Those I spoke with who had established such services in Virginia, Boston and Berkeley all opposed involuntary treatment – but wanted to fight more than one political battle at once. They were involved in mutual support with individuals with multiple problems – drug use, homelessness, a lack of money for food, mental health problems, being victims of violence – and engaged in local activism on these issues and many more.

It could be argued that this activity has dissipated energies for achieving national political rights. A spokesperson from a major professional organisation in the US told me that the radicals who used to fight psychiatric oppression were now all running drop-ins, 'which is marvellous'. One survivor activist in the US – not running services – saw two movements in operation: the 'crumb' movement ('The government is throwing us some crumbs') and the independent movement. In the UK, many activists have become user consultants, paid by mental health services; again, this may have diverted energies away from rights-based activism. Yet these activities have tested Chamberlin's early ideas for user-run alternatives, developed social and support networks for user/survivors on their own terms, and begun to influence mainstream agendas for research and service development. User-run research is growing (Faulkner 1997), and mainstream writers are acknowledging that 'consumers can bring to service encounters different attitudes, motivations, insights and behavioral qualities than can professionals' (Moxley and Mowbray 1997). At last, it seems recognised not only that user/survivors might have 'insights', but also that they may be particularly useful insights for work with others experiencing mental health problems.

If people campaign only for service developments, without opposing compulsory treatment, they may add to the sum of coercion. Equally, however, there is a danger that if a pure libertarian position prevailed, services could be left unreformed, run down and in some cases lost – perhaps for good – given continuing public expenditure controls. In the absence of support services, there might be increased incarceration in jails. For some, that is a price well worth paying for freedom from forced treatment; for others, it is not. For many, the answer is to work for both freedom from coercion and service reform.

The risks are sharpened by the fact that arguing solely against forced treatment may be ineffective. In Britain, the civil liberties position has been blamed for two things: the supposed (but not actual) rise in homicides committed by people 'released' from psychiatric hospital (Zito Trust 1997), and the cuts in mental health services, which, it is argued, were cynically justified by government via a rhetoric of expanded opportunities through 'community care' (see, for example, *Independent*, 19 January 1998, *Sunday Express*, 18 January 1998). In this context, the general public appears very hostile to libertarian arguments, which it connects with increased violence and cost cutting (see Ch. 11). It seems extremely unlikely to support any government intending to reduce coercion over user/survivors. However, members of the public do appear open to the view that users – like other disabled people – can make a contribution, for example through work (see, for instance, *The Times*, 7 June 1997), and that they need support (see Ch. 11). Strategically, it may be far more effective to argue first for citizenship participation and then to show the nonsense of Joe and Joanne – whom people now recognise as citizens who contribute – being unfairly forcibly treated. At worst, arguing only for civil liberties might lead to backsliding in other areas, from work to service reform, and no increase in civil liberties.

Further problems emerge in relation to 'reasonable accommodations' at work. While views are deeply divided on the pros and cons of disclosing mental illness and seeking accommodations (as will be explored further in Ch. 9), many user/survivors want workplaces to be made accessible to them. They do not want a model of 'responsibility' that says they must be exactly the same as people with no mental health problems in order to be accepted in the workplace. That is to fall in with the notion that the world cannot be changed – that *they* must change. It is to accept a model of 'responsibility' that is entirely defined by people who are not user/survivors (as discussed in Ch. 2) and to assume that user/survivors have to manage without support or adjustment in order to prove that they are 'responsible'. A libertarian might respond that some workplace adjustments could be achieved by the persuasion of employers, there being no need for laws to regulate relationships between individuals and businesses. For many user/survivors, however, relations with business – or lack of relations when business continually refuses to hire them – are just as critical as relations with psychiatry and the state (Rogers *et al.* 1993). A 1997 British consultation by Mind on discrimination in employment and related spheres attracted a far higher response than any previous consultations on compulsory ECT or high doses of neuroleptic drugs. There is no reason to privilege the use of law to protect citizens from the state over laws to protect them from other discriminations – other than libertarian beliefs, which in an era of relatively unaccountable global corporations overestimate the power of national governments as the oppressors of individuals.

A further critique concerns the assumption that treatment without consent is only an oppression. From the point of view of those prescribing it, it is often seen as an attempt to help someone by reducing their symptoms, symptoms that, if reduced, might enable them to make different types of choice (Grisso and Appelbaum 1998). One problem here is often a divergence in priorities between user/survivors and providers (as discussed in Ch. 4). If professionals were trained to see that user/survivors' exercise of power is as vital as symptom reduction, and that the trauma of forced treatment often can and should be avoided through advance directives or advocacy, we might attain a service governed by user/survivors' collective understandings of how best to respond to extreme distress. We might then choose to argue that the state does have a duty, as the representative of collective responsibility, to ensure that people who become extremely disturbed have a safe space and types of help that may, on the advice of the user/survivors whose ideas govern the service, provide respite. This is not to argue for treatment when someone clearly shows that they do not want it, but for engagement with the ethical dilemmas of how to 'reach out' to people in extreme distress, who may not be expressing anything clearly either way, without trampling over their preferences. Liberty alone is not a sufficient guide to how to achieve this.

Some user/survivors opposed to all forced treatment argue that treatments for physical illness could be given when someone was so distressed as to be incapacitated, even without consent – for example, if a diabetic were neither consenting to nor refusing insulin – but that the same does not apply to, for example, antidepressants. This is inconsistent. Some people, at least, would choose in advance – if given the opportunity – to take antidepressants if they became incapacitated. Withholding antidepressants from someone who had made no advance directive is essentially imposing an anti-psychiatric drugs view on those individuals, which does not fit with libertarian notions of individual choice.

A further sticking point is criminal responsibility. I put to Stephen Bright, Director of the Southern Center for Human Rights, the idea that people diagnosed as mentally ill should assume full responsibility for crime. He countered that, in California, some people who were hearing voices were set to hard labour in the fields. Unable to do the work because of the voices, they were locked down in the punishment area of the prison, in effect being punished for their mental health problems. In Alabama, a man with learning disabilities was threatened with the death penalty. Some local advocates would not oppose the execution, on the grounds that the man should take responsibility. 'With friends like that, who needs enemies? Shouldn't we be reaching out to someone who has committed a crime and has particular problems – as the native American culture does – rather than just punishing them?'

From the libertarian perspective the way to oppose forced treatment is to take total responsibility, arguing that while some people will lose out in the criminal justice system, this is ethically defensible in the light of the overall gains in civil rights. Another path would be to presume that user/survivors virtually always have total, or partial, responsibility for their crimes, but to give much more attention to mitigation where – and only where – this is relevant. That way, they might be jailed for an offence but able to keep off the chain gangs if later 'misdemeanours' were clearly the result of mental health problems. Alternatively, they might be treated through 'problem-solving policing' that took account of their own prolonged victimisation or deep poverty, as contexts for both understanding the crime and developing strategies to support them in not re-offending. This emphasis on mitigation – unlike the idea that 'mentally ill' people generally lack responsibility – does not conflict with the goal of combating compulsory treatment.

The parameters of these discussions would be different if the criminal justice system *per se* were not so punitive. The chain gangs have no purpose except humiliation: Alabama state highway officials stated that they had no need for crushed rock (Southern Center for Human Rights 1995). Clinton interrupted his 1992 campaign to oversee the execution of a man with brain damage; he refused clemency, although the man was said to be howling like a dog, and instead promised to expand the death penalty, which he subsequently did (Bright and Keenan 1995). Judges campaigning for re-election have timed death penalty cases to impact positively on their election chances; the people charged are usually poor, black and badly represented (Bright 1995).

In this climate, part of the reason for opposing the execution of juveniles or people diagnosed as mentally ill is to chip away at the death penalty when it is hard politically to oppose it outright. Similarly, in Britain, advocacy organisations argue for diversion from custody in order to extricate user/survivors from the horrors of overcrowded jails, when they might not support diversion as a matter of principle. These strategies can have the unintended effect of reaffirming in the public mind the idea that people with mental health problems are poor incompetents who cannot take responsibility.

General arguments that 'mentally ill' people should be diverted from custody, or not executed, should be abandoned in favour of arguing in specific cases for mitigation, and for 'problem-solving' approaches on a non-discriminatory basis with other citizens, which, while they may sometimes involve keeping people out of jail, do not assume that jail is 'no place for the mentally ill'.

The hospital system, too, can be highly punitive. It tends to involve indefinite sentences, which may be more hated than the most overcrowded prison regime. It too is influenced by elections and other political pressures. The pressures that psychiatrists face never to discharge someone who might later commit a violent crime are considerable – and extremely hard to fulfil without locking up all kinds of people who would never have been violent. Studies of prediction by mental health professionals of violence suggest some, but not a huge, improvement over chance (Monahan 1993). In 1997, a psychiatrist stated on British TV that he would prefer to lock up nine people who would not have committed any crime than to risk one person harming a member of the public, a particularly frank admission of the practice of incarcerating innocent people (*Panorama* 1997).

One American activist suggested to me that it was irrelevant whether people were in hospital or jail: both involved being drugged against your will and little of any value or help. Diversion from custody could therefore be something of a dead debate. In principle, however, it is important that user/survivors are seen to take responsibility and to be punished on a fair basis with other citizens. Hospitals are viewed, rightly or wrongly, as places of treatment, rather than punishment. If hospitals were used less for incarceration following crime, perhaps user/survivors too might experience them as being less punitive.

Arguing for absolute criminal responsibility, with little attention to mitigation, does have risks in a punitive climate. But so does arguing for wholesale diversion from custody, not only because it

masks the control of forced treatment as something benign, but
because it explains more and more violent crime in terms of individual pathology. By calling people 'mentally ill' by definition if
they commit certain types of crime, discrimination against everyone diagnosed as mentally ill could worsen as the label becomes
ever more strongly associated with violence. In Britain in the mid-
1990s, Marjorie Wallace argued that 100 homicides a year were
committed by mentally ill people, a figure arrived at by including
not only those whose prior mental health problems were irrelevant
to their crimes of robbery or jealousy, but also those who developed
depression in prison and were transferred to hospital as a result.
The figures became a very convenient focus for people's anxieties
about violent crime in general: it must be caused by there being
more 'madness' on the streets (Sayce 1995a).

Some experts on violence and mental disorder take great care
over how their data are reported. John Monahan, for example, has
worked with advocacy groups to plan how his work should be
used without sensationalising or exaggerating it. Others are less
responsible. Psychiatrist Dr James Grigson has given evidence in
death penalty cases on whether someone found guilty is likely to
kill again. Usually on the basis of meeting the person once, he has
claimed accurate predictive ability. In one case, the person he
asserted would kill again went on to be absolved of the crime altogether – but he stood his ground and reasserted that this man
would 'kill again'. Grigson became known for persuasive abilities
with juries. For example, on seeing that one jury member was
reluctant to believe that a man should die, he discovered she had a
14-year-old daughter and worked with the prosecution to bring up
the question of whether the defendant would be likely to murder
14-year-old girls. In this case – and many others – the jury voted
unanimously for execution (Rosenbaum 1990). This doctor was
discredited by the APA but continued to practise.

In this instance, psychiatric diagnosis is used not to show that
people need to be diverted from custody or otherwise treated
'softly', but rather to define people as sociopaths, abnormal people
who should therefore be treated more harshly. Their 'abnormality'
means not that they should be treated equally under the law, as
Williams wants, but that they should be killed precisely because
their pathology means that there is a probability that they will
commit acts of violence which would constitute a continuing threat
to society, one of the standards that has to be met, for example, for
executions in Texas (Rosenbaum 1990). This particular trend is

more common in the US – which tends more to the punitive than to the patronising model of forensic psychiatry – than in the UK. In arguing that user/survivors should take responsibility, it is important for advocates not inadvertently to give ammunition to those wishing to explain violence in terms of madness, nor to those arguing that people with 'mental illness' deserve harsher punishment than others.

Conclusion

None of the above analysis constitutes a critique of the goal of securing an end to discriminatory laws that permit the compulsory treatment and detention of people with mental health problems on different grounds than for other citizens. An anti-discrimination agenda must include the repeal of discriminatory laws. It does question, however, whether this is the only priority. It does so from a very European perspective, which sees rights and responsibilities in social rather than purely individual terms.

The core of this approach is that responsibility is shared – it is not all held by government on the one hand or by the individual on the other. In a sense, we are all responsible – through democratic means, through our own actions – for creating a society that does not discriminate on mental health grounds. The terrible risk with the current individualised debate on rights and responsibilities is that it argues that the individual user/survivor, in order to have any rights, has to be 100% responsible for working, fitting in, not committing crimes or making a nuisance of any kind, with little or no reciprocal responsibility on business, educational institutions, the courts or other bodies to provide opportunities or even act fairly. Rather than some user/survivors or advocates wanting rights without responsibilities, as has sometimes been claimed (see Ch. 2), we could see society at large wanting rights (to have nothing to do with people with mental health problems, to get them out of their neighbourhoods and workplaces) and still expecting user/survivors to take total responsibility. This is an unfair loading: why should users be model citizens when they are excluded from citizenship at every turn?

Arguing for social responsibility in a context of anti-discrimination principles does not mean a return to paternalistic models of welfare. Instead, it means combining individual rights with a particular insistence on responsibility from those players with significant power.

That includes the state – for if there is no change in discriminatory laws on compulsion, why should users trust the state on any measures it takes? It also includes, however, other powerful bodies, from employers to insurers.

The libertarian model has made a major contribution in highlighting abuses by the state and limiting the extension of compulsory treatment. But getting the state off users' individual backs does not seem, to many user/survivors in Britain or the US, to be a sufficient strategy. There may not be a sufficient power base to make libertarianism a strong force.

Other social movements have their libertarian wing. Andrew Sullivan argues that gay people should concentrate their campaigns on getting rid of government discrimination, in sodomy laws, marriage laws and access to the military, rather than dealing with 'private' discrimination by companies and individuals (Sullivan 1995). However, the lesbian and gay communities have successfully negotiated dilemmas very similar to those of the mental health movement, including wanting services from the same government that is seen as oppressive. Since the advent of AIDS, they have found ways of arguing both for 'getting the government out of the bedroom' and for obtaining government funds, and have pushed for anti-discrimination provisions in work, insurance and other areas of 'private' life. None of these approaches appears to have undermined the others. And – exactly as in mental health – the call for laws opposing unfair discrimination in housing, employment and the like is known to stand a much higher chance of public support than are purely libertarian arguments (Vaid 1995, see also Ch. 11).

Pursuing several fronts at once is nonetheless inevitably complex and fraught with contention in terms of the order of priorities and how to avoid the dissipation of energies (as we shall see in the next chapter). The pure libertarian model provides a clear answer: oppose forced treatment. Many other strands of user/survivor activism, and disability activism, have, however, formulated more multifaceted answers, which set the agenda slightly differently. The next chapter explores these wider approaches to increasing social inclusion.

CHAPTER 7

The Disability Inclusion Model: No to Shame

The disability inclusion model aims to dismantle the discrimination faced by people because they have a diagnosis or record of mental illness, and to open up new opportunities. It does not matter where the discrimination occurs: in the legal system, the hospital ward, the boss's office or the TV studio. The constructions of user/survivors as morally tainted, dangerous, to be feared and segregated, have to be replaced and the discriminatory behaviour of employers, judges and 'nimby' campaigners curbed. The aim is citizenship inclusion, on a fair basis with all other citizens – and fairness for would-be citizens, who should not be barred from immigration on the grounds of mental disorder. This would change user/survivors' lived experience – people's income, opportunities and legal rights – rather than only, as in the 'brain disease' and 'individual growth' models, making it easier for people to seek help. The paternalistic notion that all disabled people need is 'services' to 'help' them has to be replaced by a broader view of people's aspirations and potential.

This is a civil rights, as opposed to a civil libertarian, agenda. It is about positive rights – to fair opportunities and, for some, adjustments/supports to make them viable – as well as negative rights, to be free of unfair coercion.

Its direct challenge to discrimination – legal, institutional and attitudinal – leads this approach straight into the broader disability movement's civil rights agenda. The social model of disability – which says that people are disabled not, or not only, by their so-called 'impairment' (that is, physical, mental or emotional difference from the norm), but instead by the barriers and prejudices that society places in their way – becomes a banner under which user/survivors and other disabled people can rally. 'Attitudes are the real disability', as one movement car sticker put it. Discrimination must be torn away, not only that committed by government (as in the libertarian model), but also that by employers, schools, shops and all other organisations. In addition, positive steps must be taken to improve access, for example, making a company's services accessible to deaf people by providing minicom services, and making workplaces accessible by offering individualised accommodations such as extra feedback for someone who experiences anxiety, so that they can do their job effectively.

User/survivors and other disabled people all share discrimination on the basis of some presumed 'imperfection' of body, mind or emotion and can join together in challenging the very idea of perfection. Together they can tackle the common experience of massive exclusion – albeit on the basis of different stereotypes (the tragic blind person, the heroic wheelchair user succeeding against the odds or the violent 'psycho-killer'; Pointon and Davies 1997).

In this model, disability activists have mobilised across the US to achieve access for disabled students on campuses, a deaf president for the deaf university Gallaudet, and eventually civil rights laws to outlaw discrimination against disabled people generally (Shapiro 1993). The mental health user/survivor movement has more recently joined forces in a growing movement for full and enforced civil rights. Even in Britain's limited Disability Discrimination Act 1995, survivors' needs were to an extent covered: for example, Mind lobbied successfully to ensure that people with 'personality disorder' had some protection. Also, British mental health rehabilitation specialists have used the concept of 'disability' as a basis on which to develop work and social opportunities for people with mental health problems (Wing and Morris 1981, Perkins and Repper 1996).

Survivor activist Judi Chamberlin has travelled the US facilitating greater links between survivors and the wider disability movement, for example encouraging Independent Living Centers to be inclusive of user/survivors of mental health services (Chamberlin 1995). She describes her own learning experience:

Almost all the problems that persons with physical disabilities face are shared by persons with psychiatric disabilities (for example difficulty in accessing housing, employment, and community services)... we have grown closer to the disability community and discovered the commonalities that we share. In the beginning this was difficult for both communities because there were mutual levels of mistrust and of feeling that we did not have the same problems. Many people with physical disabilities feared being lumped in with 'crazy' people, while many former mental patients took the position that 'We're not disabled, we're just oppressed'... What has happened has been a process of mutual unlearning in which persons with both physical and psychiatric disabilities have learnt to undo stereotypes and myths and to see each other as the individuals we are (Chamberlin 1993).

In the UK, alliances are newer and more fragile, but by 1997, the Greater London Association of Disabled People had held a conference on mental health issues; the government's Task Force on civil rights for disabled people included mental health representation; and David Grayson, Chair of the National Disability Council, stated on BBC radio that disabled people – including people with mental health problems (the first on his list) – faced highly discriminatory imagery in the media. Cross-disability thinking was beginning to develop in the UK.

The disability rights model places user/survivors as a minority group in society – like black British people or African Americans – but it also acknowledges the huge intersections between different lines of difference: many people are African American users or have other complex triple or quadruple-barrelled identities. It aims to learn from other civil rights movements' experiences and not to expect people to leave one identity – say, being a woman – at the door in order to join a male-dominated user organisation. It aims to practise what it preaches in relation to inclusion and to address issues of discrimination faced by, for example, deaf people who are part of the user/survivor movement (Gifford *et al.* 1996). Vernon (1995) has argued powerfully for addressing 'simultaneous' rather than 'double' or 'triple' discrimination within the disability movement; it is not an additive matter, but one of complex interactions between different discriminations. Also, it is not a minority concern: most disabled people are not white, middle-class men 'but rather... disabled working-class men, women, gays and lesbians, older people and people of Irish, Jewish and many other ethnic origins'.

Attempts are made within at least some disability organisations to learn about each other's experiences of discrimination, so that, for example, user/survivors do not undermine other disabled people by arguing that they should have access to work because they are 'able-bodied' or 'not stupid', and those with learning difficulties do not say that they should be free of discrimination because they are 'not crazy'.

In the UK, the Women and Mental Health Forum worked with Justice for Women in 1997 to highlight the intersection of discriminations on gender and mental health grounds in the case of Josie O'Dwyer. O'Dwyer killed a man who, she alleged, tried to rape her, but she changed her plea from manslaughter to murder at the last minute in court, partly for fear of being 'nutted off' – sent for an indefinite sentence to a secure hospital – and partly because she had just learnt for the first time in court that she had been sexually assaulted in childhood and was probably in shock. Josie O'Dwyer committed suicide in prison before justice could be obtained for her, but activists continued to campaign both for more understanding in the judicial system of the impact of rape, in both childhood and adulthood, and for a radical change in the way in which secure hospitals operate for women.

Within the disability inclusion model, user/survivors have begun to frame the type of support they want in terms of a 'disability' analysis. The growing 'recovery' movement – promoted through recovery groups and recovery workbooks, which encourage people to take stock and set new life paths – provides a vision of moving from the despair of very changed circumstances on becoming a 'user' to hope. The hope is not about 'cure' but about leading a fulfilling life with mental health problems, which are valued as part of experience. Patricia Deegan puts it this way:

> Recovery does not refer to an end-product or result. It does not mean that my friend [with quadriplegia] and I were 'cured'. In fact, our recovery is marked by an ever-deepening acceptance of our limitations. But now, rather than being an occasion for despair, we find that our personal limitations are the ground from which spring our own unique possibilities (Deegan 1994a).

This process of recovery can only work if the external environment enables people to develop 'their own unique possibilities'. Recovery is totally dependent on civil rights and opportunities for inclusion. They are congruent belief systems, both based on valuing people who are different and not just those who 'fit in'. Sometimes the 'recovery' movement veers a little more into cure-based 'individual growth' notions, as when it gets overly linked with the concept of 'recovery' used in 12-step programmes, to mean a requirement for self-improvement (see Ch. 5). Bureau (1993) notes that 'the language of AA's version of recovery is seductive, but we are not addicted to it. Not yet.' Generally, however, the wider recovery movement offers the possibility of finding a new ground for being, one that does not require a person to 'grow' into the total health of someone else's formulation.

'We're not disabled': a central critique of disability rights

Many user/survivors do not wish to embrace the disability model. There is considerable concern at the prospect of being 'incorporated' into the disability movement, which, critics argue, has always neglected mental distress alongside other 'unpopular' impairments such as AIDS and illegal drug use. The key historical text on the disability movement, *No Pity* by Shapiro (1993), not only neglects the history of the mental health movement – something Williams describes as a typical attempt to ensure that 'our bad odor will not rub off on the respectable disabilities' (Williams X 1995) – but also cites only one individual with a mental health problem, who abuses the person in his care. Thus are user/survivors stereotyped even within disability rights thinking.

Many user/survivors resist defining themselves as 'disabled' for a number of reasons. A seminar for European user/survivors in 1994 revealed varying views on the term 'disability', and considerable concern (European Network of Users and Ex-users of Psychiatry 1994). Sayce (1998b), however, questions whether some of these reasons are based on misconceptions about what 'disability' means, for example:

- Disabled people (some user/survivors believe) have a tangible impairment, for example, being unable to walk or see. A diagnosis of mental illness is much more in the eye of the beholder; it is not clear that there is something 'wrong'.

People in the disability rights movement challenge the idea that there is a norm of perfection against which they are judged to have an 'impairment', just as survivors do (Shapiro 1993, Morris 1996). Many in the deaf movement consider themselves to be a linguistic minority with their own positive culture. Historically, the words 'impairment' and 'disability' have carried the negative connotations of having something 'wrong' and being 'unable', but activists have reclaimed the terms under the social model of disability. One can be 'disabled' and positively different – exactly as one can be 'mad and proud' (as discussed in Ch. 1).

● The only thing that disables user/survivors is the way in which society excludes and stigmatises them. Otherwise they are not disabled.

The 'social model' of disability has space for people who believe that it is only the barriers erected by society that 'disable' people, for example, 'it is not a problem to me that I have no legs. My only problem is the fact that society denies me access to places because of its attitudes and the way it has built cities and buildings' (disabled activist, Washington DC, 1996). Increasingly, however, some disabled people, especially feminists, have argued that the impact of the impairment itself has been underestimated. For example:

> Do we believe that admitting there could be a difficult side to impairment will undermine the strong, positive (Supercrip) images of our campaigns?... Or even that admitting it can sometimes be awful to have impairments may fuel the belief that our lives are not worth living?... The experience of impairment is not always irrelevant... How can it be when pain, fatigue, depression and chronic illness are constant facts of life for many of us? (Crow 1996).

Under the social model, user/survivors who believe that mental illness is a construct used to discriminate can be included. So can those who believe that 'madness' is positive and life-enhancing. And so can those, like Liz Crow, who think that 'impairment' itself – being so depressed that one cannot function, or terrified by persecutory voices – is truly problematic but cannot be separated from the discrimination that compounds the 'impairment' at every turn.

● Mental distress is not a disability because it is not something that you are born with and it is not permanent; people recover, they are 'survivors'.

Most people with physical and sensory impairments are not born that way; they acquire disability, through accidents and late-onset problems, compounded by discrimination and exclusion. In 1991–92, only 5.2% of Americans under 18 years of age were disabled compared with 13.6% of 18–44-year-olds, 29.2% of 45–64-year-olds, 44.6% of 65–74-year-olds, 63.7% of 75–84-year-olds and 84.2% of people aged 85 and above (McNeil 1993). As with mental distress, there can be many social causes of the impairment, such as a lack of safety at work. There are many different patterns of impairment. Some people have episodic problems like multiple sclerosis (just as some have episodes of depression). It is impossible to generalise that physical disability is permanent. Also, for some user/survivors, problems are long-lasting; if we define mental distress as non-permanent, are we not in danger of suggesting that users' lives have value because many 'recover' or 'survive'? Where does that leave those whose lives are coloured by unremitting difficulties? It would be contrary to disability pride, or 'mad pride', to suggest that user/survivors' lives have value because they can keep one foot in the world of 'normality.'

● Disability sounds very severe. In the mental health world we want to engage the 1 in 4 people with experience of distress each year and not just those with serious diagnoses.

The same debate goes on in other disability sectors. Blindness organisations often want to engage those with any visual impairment, deafness organisations those with any hearing impairment. The social model of disability encourages a very broad movement, encompassing everyone who is liable to face discrimination because they are deemed not to be 'normal' physically, mentally or emotionally.

● Taking on the term 'disability' means taking on another stigma. Having one stigma is bad enough.

When the mental health community works with the wider disability movement to improve disability rights law, we implicitly or explicitly ask disabled people to stand firm in the face of attempts by politicians to 'pick off' mental health and other 'unpopular' groups, which means sharing in the stigma of mental illness. Working collaboratively involves coming to understand each other's experiences and sharing in the differing effects of our discriminations.

These rationales for user/survivors rejecting the concept of 'disability' are not fully convincing. However, there are major differences between mental distress and physical or sensory disability. For example:

> Unlike people with physical disabilities whose angry indignation is seen as an appropriate response to an unjust situation, our anger is often viewed as but one more symptom of our psychopathology. Indeed, many of us have learnt that we get punished for expressing our

anger, that is, our medications may be increased... we may be asked to leave a program... Learning that it is OK to be angry, that we have a lot to be angry about, that we do not have to view our anger as a symptom of mental illness, and that we do not have to accept punishment for being angry is a fundamental task... In our anger we reclaim our right to say: 'The injustice, the abuse, the degradation, and the discrimination that I have suffered is wrong. I am a valuable human being. I do not accept the conditions of oppression to which I am supposed to 'adjust' (Deegan 1994b).

It is critical that each disability group raises consciousness about the particular ways in which the group is stereotyped and excluded, and takes action to reduce discrimination. The user/survivor movement can only ensure that discrimination on mental health grounds is fully explored, understood and challenged by organising separately. However, it also has much to gain from a wider movement:

Cross-disability means to acknowledge the autonomy and celebrate the diversity of each culture of people with disabilities, while also rejecting the false barriers that are forced upon us due to our respective labels. When we join together we are the largest minority group in the country and, as the passage of the ADA proves, within our numbers we have the collective power to overcome oppression (Deegan 1994b).

While the disability movement has not always been prepared to challenge 'populist' mental health policies, notably compulsory treatment, US and UK activists have begun to use the opportunity of disability rights discussions at government level to raise the issue and to gain support from other disability leaders. In 1998, Rights Now, the British disability lobby group, supported the mental health movement in opposing a proposed extension of compulsory treatment.

User/survivors could go much further – by defining the basis of the conceptual renewal needed to free user/survivors from discrimination, and then sharing ideas with other disabled people. This would enrich the thinking of the movement as a whole. Current overarching thinking on disability rights can miss the point for user/survivors. Disabled people want rights, not pity. The pathetic image of the poster child has been thrown out along with telethons and patronising attitudes: 'Piss on pity', ran one movement headline (Hartman and Johnson 1993). For user/survivors, however, the phenomenon of the poster child, the pathetic tug at the heart strings, is not the key problem. Rather, it is being demonised, treated with fear and loathing (as described in Ch. 3).

In 1996, when One in Eight, the British disability media watch group, awarded raspberries to the most stigmatising media coverage, the 'winners' covering mobility and sensory impairments included Children In Need, a classic pitiable TV fundraiser. The one 'winner' depicting psychiatric disability was a TV drama featuring a mentally ill serial killer.

The broad disability movement rises above certain particular experiences of being shamed – as tragic, not 'body beautiful', lacking in physical prowess. The challenge for user/survivors is to overthrow a shame with a different edge to it: the explicit or implicit link to moral wrongdoing (see Ch. 3). The task is not to subvert the 'individual tragedy' notion, which Oliver (1990) sees as the defining construction of disabled identity, but to subvert the sense of moral shame.

If Shapiro (1993) had explored constructions of mental illness, and the ways in which the user/survivor movement works to challenge them, he might have concluded that 'No pity' was not a broad enough banner for an inclusive disability rights movement. 'No to shame' could be. It challenges the whole notion that shame should be attached to not fitting some notion of perfection of body, or mind, or emotion. It confronts directly the sense of moral taint that seems to float around every discussion of mental illness. It tackles the humiliation of pity alongside all other disempowering attitudes. Within this construction, people with learning disabilities who raise children could challenge the idea that they are themselves always childlike, people using wheelchairs the notion that they are tragically 'wheelchair bound' and people with mental health problems that they are dangerous to children.

The potential weakness in the slogan 'No to shame' is that it could be seen to focus on the disabled person's sense of shame – something they should change – rather than on its source, the culture's tendency to humiliate and 'shame' them. When a British mental health group came up with the draft slogan 'Stuff stigma' in planning an anti-discrimination campaign in 1997, the mood was one of combat, the aim not to adjust internal self-perceptions but to challenge the whole idea that stigma is an internal matter, to take action to tackle every type of unfair treatment. 'No to shame' could be used similarly, to mean that people will no longer put up with being shamed, nor with accepting, compliantly, that they should themselves feel ashamed, nor with the presumption that the problem lies in their psychology (see the Introduction for a fuller discussion of the risks of victim-blaming).

Shame is different from guilt. People feel guilty about things they have done; they feel ashamed of what they are, of an aspect of their identities. Shame sometimes pervades a person's life. It is usually hard to find an ethical basis for shame about an identity of any kind, as an identity may be chosen, like being a Mormon or a feminist (in which case, do you really feel shame at your chosen path? Why choose it, if part of you disagrees with it so profoundly?). Alternatively, an identity is something that is fixed, at least for the moment, by how society categorises differences, like being black, or being blind, or having serious mental health problems (in which case, why feel ashamed, when you have so little power to change the way in which you are slotted into these categories? And how can moral good or bad be relevant when there are no chosen adverse consequences – how can it be shameful to be blind or distressed?).

We may sometimes want to object, on moral grounds, to an identity that someone else has chosen – their religious or political affiliation perhaps – although, even then, we usually accept they should not face discrimination, for example, in employment. Sayce (1997b) argues that it is vital to protect users of illegal drugs from discrimination, even though they may have 'chosen' to take them: people should only be refused a job if they cannot do the job, not because someone else objects to their moral behaviour or religious practices outside work. But people do not choose to have mental health problems. Not only should they not be refused jobs when they can do them, but there is also no basis for anyone to object morally to their identity as user/survivors. There is quite simply no basis for shame.

When a person feels shame, it is worth questioning closely whether he or she actually believes in the basis for it or whether it is rather the shame of victimhood, the taint that follows being treated or described as inferior. For someone with mental health problems, shame may arise from being treated as less than a citizen (see Ch. 3), and users have written about the shame that can follow compulsory treatment:

> I found the imposition of a major tranquillizer, administered against my will in injection form on a number of occasions, very destructive to my self-confidence and integrity as a person. There are clear similarities

between the experience and accounts I've read of rape – the shame and feeling 'I must have been to blame' (quoted in Cobb 1993).

Having mental health problems is not a moral matter; how one behaves is. Key strategies for throwing off the impact of discrimination are therefore to 'come out' – visibly to refuse to be shamed just for being a user/survivor – and simultaneously to take responsibility for one's actions (see Ch. 6): to be quite prepared to feel guilty, to take the consequences, of actions that may be unethical.

If user/survivors become ever more involved in the wider disability movement, they could contribute to new overarching ideas, such as 'No to shame', which go much further than 'No pity', which challenge, ever more trenchantly, society's tendency to humiliate those it has deemed 'imperfect'.

Further critiques and counter-critiques

There are several other criticisms of the disability rights model.

First, it generates an agenda that is so massive that it could enable advocacy organisations to duck the hard and controversial issues, like forced treatment, and to 'select' safer civil rights issues on which to campaign. This could mean no effective challenge to the 'equivalent of slavery' (see Ch. 6) for a very long time.

It is certainly true that many mental health organisations have chosen to put their energies into improving employment opportunities under various 'welfare-to-work' schemes, or into managed care and other health policy issues, rather than into opposing compulsory treatment. However, it is by no means clear that organisations that take more moderate positions somehow 'undermine' those seeking far-reaching change. Studies of the environmental movement suggest that the 'no compromise' approach of Earth First is directly complementary to mainstream environmental activities. Earth First obtains media coverage of the issue through dramatic media stunts; they act as a foil, their extremism rendering other environmentalists positively attractive to politicians by comparison, and they transform the debate within the environmental movement (Lange 1990).

Similarly, in the American mental health world, the focus on combating compulsory ECT by Support Coalition International, and the intellectually powerful and uncompromising anti-compulsion arguments of libertarian activists, change the terms of debate. At the same time, as user/survivors obtain more civil rights through cross-disability work, pushed by survivor activists and more mainstream organisations, the effort to abolish or reduce compulsory treatment could become easier. It is harder compulsorily to treat people who have become workers, parents and respected citizens. The efforts are potentially complementary.

The second objection to the disability model is that a pluralistic agenda may mean that the pursuit of one aim, such as parity between mental and physical health care, cuts across the objectives of another, such as combating forced treatment. Parity means more treatment, which means more forced treatment. Both issues are clear-cut cases of discrimination. Views differ on which is a higher priority. Some user/survivors have campaigned for parity: indeed, one public demonstration in Philadelphia targeted a private sector company, Blue Cross Blue Shield, in a relatively unusual example of activism targeting a corporation. User/survivors in Philadelphia have also demonstrated in favour of a properly resourced, single-stream-funded managed care service for mental health – and, when it was under threat, entered the Capital building to protest. The Governor's 'I shall have order' statements were met each time by the response 'We shall have disorder', until the user/survivor organisation won its case (Rogers, personal communication 1997).

There is no simple way of avoiding conflicts between objectives. The world is complex. Campaigning strategies have to address this complexity by trying to predict unintended consequences, thinking creatively about ways of avoiding negative impact and communicating with other groups to try to make actions complementary. Common ground may be found, for example, through a campaign explicitly demanding more voluntary services. Even where advocates disagree profoundly, if one group achieves a high profile for a mental health issue, another may be able to capitalise on the attention to make a different argument.

The third problem is that a very broad agenda simply dissipates energies and waters down effectiveness. This is why, for example, Support Coalition International in 1996/97 focused not even on combating compulsory treatment but on combating the 'force and fraud' of compulsory electroshock. People need to concentrate on winnable objectives. In 1996, the organisation's 1000 members knew the priority and were enabled to do something about it through Internet advice on lobbying, monthly 'tea parties' and the provision of materials. David Oakes, a leader in Support Coalition, believed that there were many other priorities too: for example, making alliances with disability groups and labour unions, and healing 'normality' – defined in terms of being 'nice' to people even when you can't stand them (diagnosed as inappropriate smiling), being serious – never playful or creative (stiff upper lippity), being obedient (adjustment prone), cool (tearlessnicity) and boring (hyperinactivity) (Foner 1997). Pursuing all these priorities at once, however, would mean being ineffectual.

While running a single-issue campaign, one can hold a vision of more major change, otherwise the focus on a short-term winnable issue acts as a set of blinkers. In 1992–94, Mind ran a UK campaign focusing on four issues of concern to women, one of which, the need for safety in hospital settings, took priority. The campaign achieved some successes: providing a space in which many women spoke for the first time about assault in psychiatric wards; enabling women to make complaints; raising public awareness through the mass media; gaining support from key politicians; influencing professional bodies publicly to support choice for women of being on a single-sex ward; and achieving some change in national and local policy. The campaign was, however, conducted within a framework of a much broader set of policy aims, which included influencing parental rights decisions and setting up more non-hospital services for women. It would have been highly problematic to concentrate only on changing hospital wards and forget longer-term goals like enabling some women to avoid hospitalisation in the first place (Sayce 1995b).

Within the disability rights model, single-issue campaigns are essential, but one issue should not determine the agenda. One single issue should follow another, or occur alongside another, as different groups inevitably select different priorities. A broad agenda also enables a movement to be flexible. In Britain in 1997, a new government brought opportunities to influence civil rights law and welfare-to-work schemes as they affected user/survivors. At that moment, achievements in these areas were in prospect – if the opportunity was seized – whereas reductions in coercive treatment were much less likely, given the calls from many quarters for increased controls. Advocates sought to advance policy on civil rights, at the same time as undertaking damage limitation in relation to coercion. Concentrating only on coercion would probably have meant no gains at all; focusing only on civil rights would have meant substantial losses in relation to compulsory treatment. A broad agenda provides space for tactical decisions.

The fourth problem is that arguing for greater 'opportunity' means giving people the chance to succeed or fail in the lottery of life – and some will fail. Some will end up 'dying with their rights on'. What is instead needed is a commitment to equality – of outcome, not of opportunity. This argument has some pertinence in relation to the most marginalised groups (as will be discussed in Ch. 9). However, opportunity is on offer in market economies; absolute equality is not. Some user/survivors can benefit if, and only if, mental health advocates ensure that users' needs are fed into plans for civil rights law, support to get and keep jobs, and other opportunities. At the same time, mental health organisations can work in coalition with other groups of marginalised people – such as poverty and older people's groups – to highlight the way in which some people are still left wholly excluded and disenfranchised.

The fifth problem is that arguing for 'civil rights' may risk a 'backlash'. The public is in no mood for yet another 'minority group' seeking 'special rights'. The difficulty with this argument is that the 'backlash' is in truth a forelash (see Ch. 10). It may be that the more meek and mild the mental health world becomes, the more – not less – it will be trampled by groups with their own agenda: free marketeers who object to civil rights law, those in favour of genetic screening to reduce the number of disabled people or those advocating more controls through electronic tagging. Users/survivors and allies need to stand firm and simultaneously explain the aims of inclusion in ways that will be understood. The public may assume that 'rights' mean the civil libertarian right to be free of compulsory detention. They may wrongly believe that this means people would be able to commit crimes with impunity. It is important to convey that this is a movement of people who want to contribute and who seek responsibilities and fair opportunities to be included in social and economic life. In Europe, where the concept of civil rights has so much less resonance than in the US, it is especially useful to talk in the language of active citizenship.

Conclusion

Given the continuing segregation faced by user/survivors, bolstered by ideas of moral degradation, the highest priority for the next major stage of development is to overturn that central core of discriminatory thinking and behaviour (as described in

Ch. 3). Of all the models currently adopted to tackle 'stigma' or discrimination, the one that holds most promise is the disability inclusion model. It does not contain within it seeds of discriminatory ideas. It neither removes all responsibility from user/survivors (see Ch. 4), nor makes them responsible for being 'mentally ill' (Ch. 5), nor makes their rights dependent on responsibly 'fitting in', with no reciprocal obligation on powerful bodies in society (Ch. 6). It assumes that user/survivors are responsible, in a context of the wider responsibilities of society to break apart the barriers of discrimination. With political will, in time, this model could bring new and more equal relationships between user/survivors and other citizens.

The brain disease, individual growth and libertarian models are not entirely without potential to assist in achieving this goal. Libertarian challenges to compulsory treatment are an essential aspect of the struggle for civil rights, and campaigns aiming to encourage more people to seek help – be it medical, psychological or spiritual – can at least lift the taboo on discussing mental distress. Users and advocates can sometimes ride on the back of well-funded 'seek help' campaigns: once stigma is established in the public mind as a problem, it is a small step to inform people of the realities of discrimination, as Mind did by publishing surveys in 1996 and 1997, to huge media response (Read and Baker 1996, Repper *et al.* 1997).

But these three models are limited. Cyclical analysts attribute the repeated 'failure' of big ideas in mental health policy to the fact that their proponents did not address the complexity of factors influencing the particular policy advocated. The future social position of user/survivors will be affected by everything from economic policy to subtle shifts in cultural attitudes. The disability inclusion model is able to address this: by objecting to discrimination wherever it occurs, from the government committee report to the conversation in a bar, and by forging multiple alliances, being flexible, selecting single issues tactically to achieve greatest effect.

The disability inclusion model is highly inclusive. It can accommodate people seeking healing or cure, through any means from chanting to Prozac, but being 'healed' or 'in recovery' is quite unnecessary to being in this change movement, which explicitly values people whether they 'recover' or not. There is, in addition, no need to commit oneself to a particular understanding of 'mental illness' and no orthodoxy stating that one should feel guilty for not taking psychiatric drugs, or – as can happen in some survivor environments – for taking them. The disability rights model can sit alongside beliefs that there should be more talking treatments, or none at all.

This approach is driven neither by the particular vested interests of companies selling products nor by family members seeking explanations that do not blame them. It is derived from user/survivors' experiences of discrimination – which are unacceptable for them, and costly for society (as we saw in Ch. 1). Family members and friends may gain from this model, which could reduce the 'shame' of being associated with someone who is 'mentally ill'. Also, the appeal to justice could begin to make those not directly affected see – as colleagues, neighbours and potential friends – that access for people with mental health problems is an issue affecting everyone.

One might find that a 'No to shame' banner would also appeal to mental health professionals, who, like relatives, can pick up discriminatory attitudes at one remove: why on earth, they may be asked at parties, work with 'crazy' people, of all things? Alliances between user/survivors and professionals would, however, coalesce around user/survivors' interests rather than around a market-driven campaign for more people to seek help, geared to boosting sales or helping a provider's case for additional grants.

Through cross-disability work, user/survivors may gradually begin to count on the support of other disabled people, as the common experience of being excluded and shamed becomes better recognised. Alliances with other groups – such as black and minority groups and women's groups – could ensure that multiple discrimination was simultaneously addressed. The separate organisation and strength of the user/survivor movement could be complemented by a range of new allies.

The disability incusion model has also begun to be translated into practice through major legislative and policy change, as we shall see in the next chapter.

CHAPTER 8

The Potential of
Anti-discrimination Law

Once we have established a clear aim of working for social inclusion and developed banner headlines like 'No to shame', 'Full participation', even 'Mad and proud' – to replace hate, to head off pity – we are still left with the crunch question of how best to achieve change.

The disability rights movement's most fundamental goal has been comprehensive, and fully enforced, civil rights law. In the mental health movement, some have concentrated more on public education: if only, the argument goes, people understood more about mental health, prejudices would fall away. These positions beg fundamental questions about what exactly alters people's thoughts and behaviour. Does law stop people discriminating even where it is ahead of public opinion – when attitudes have not 'caught up'? How do we avoid public education messages that people dismiss out of hand – or alternatively that alter attitudes, but leave behaviour untouched? Health educationalists may have convinced most of us that exercise is good for health, but this does not automatically rouse us from our armchairs.

In the next few chapters, I examine the successes and potential of different methods used to date: anti-discrimination law, public and political debate, media and arts-based work to influence public opinion and grassroots projects to achieve inclusion. I begin with the potential, and limitations, of law.

The 1990 ADA is widely regarded as the world's most comprehensive disability discrimination law (Bynoe *et al.*, 1991 West 1996) (see Ch. 9 for international comparisons). Is a law of this kind the solution to discrimination on mental health grounds?

The ADA is a civil rights law, aiming to remove the historical exclusion of people with disabilities. It provides protections from discrimination and improved access for people who have a disability, a history of a disability or a perceived disability in fields including employment, access to public services, public accommodations, private services and telecommunications. A disability is defined as a physical or mental impairment that substantially limits one or more major life activities.

All employers with 15 employees or more are debarred from discriminating against a 'qualified' disabled individual. They also have to make reasonable accommodations (called reasonable adjustments under UK law) for qualified individuals in the workplace, such as providing extra support or a quiet space to work for someone with mental health problems, unless this would cause 'undue hardship' (for example, if a technological accommodation, like computer equipment, were too costly for a small company to bear).

In services and accommodations ranging from concert halls to transportation, discrimination on grounds of disability is banned, and structural changes have to be made (on a phased basis) to provide access, provided that this is 'readily achievable'. Unsurprisingly, the definitions of terms such as 'undue hardship' and 'readily achievable' have been subject to much testing in the courts. For a general explanation of the provisions of the Act, see Gooding (1994); for an explanation in relation to psychiatric disability, see Mental Health Law Project (1992) and Rubenstein (1993).

The law's coverage of psychiatric disability is gradually becoming more prominent. In 1997, the Equal Employment Opportunity Commission (EEOC) – which covers disability, race and gender discrimination – issued Enforcement Guidance on the ADA and psychiatric disability, which stated unequivocally that many people face employment discrimination because their psychiatric disabilities 'are stigmatised or misunderstood': it also reported that Congress intended the ADA to combat this discrimination 'as well as the myths, fears and stereotypes upon which it is based' (Equal Employment Opportunity Commission 1997).

Successive pieces of EEOC Guidance have defined which 'life activities' are substantially limited by impairments in ways that constitute 'disability'. The list now includes concentrating, interacting with others, learning, thinking and sleeping – where previously the examples all pertained to physical or sensory activities, such as walking and seeing. The Guidance explains how 'limited' a person has to be in these areas in order to be considered disabled. Some unfriendliness with co-workers would not constitute a substantial limitation in interacting with others. Regular, severe problems would. The EEOC cites a young man with a diagnosis of schizophrenia who, prior to treatment, stayed in his room for months, usually refusing to talk to friends and close family. Being covered by the ADA, he obtained work following treatment and functioned successfully as a computer programmer in a large company (Equal Employment Opportunity Commission 1997). Episodic impairments, such as recurrent depression, are covered, along with more continuous long-term impairments.

The ADA built on and extended previous disability law, notably the Rehabilitation Act 1973, which banned discrimination by the federal government and agencies contracted by government. Some states also had disability discrimination laws predating the ADA, and Fair Housing law was making some, albeit constrained, headway in debarring housing discrimination (Allen 1996). A city like Washington DC, with many federal agencies, thus already had 20 years' experience of improving disability access when the ADA came into force. Its metro system is used by wheelchair users – unlike London's underground; ticket machines have instructions in Braille; and on the train, announcements – transmitted from near the door to enable blind passengers to follow the sound – specify which side of the train the doors will open. Many huge barriers persist, in Washington and across the US, but in some respects progress is beyond the dreams of many British disabled citizens. The ADA built from this success. For example, between 1989 and 1994, bus fleet accessibility increased from 36% to 50% (West 1996).

The Rehabilitation Act is also credited with bringing new ideas about disability to disabled people themselves, through a training programme run by and for disabled people. The result, according to Mary Lou Breslin, President of Disability Rights Education and Defense Fund (DREDF), was that 'people saw for the first time that the problem wasn't them, for being unable to walk into a building – it was the building, for having steps. It was a completely new way of looking at the world. It led to a quiet revolution, for instance people with developmental disabilities and their parents lobbying successfully for independent housing – not group homes, but their own housing' (Breslin, personal communication, 1996).

However, this quiet revolution did not significantly include mental health user/survivors at this point. From 1985–90, only 564 complaints of discrimination against people with mental health problems were received in EEOC offices compared with 4449 pertaining to physical disability (Moss 1991).

The question is, has the ADA forged new ground? As to whether the ADA promises positive change generally, opinions differ wildly:

> Our success will support the emancipation of millions of people in the 21st century in America and across the world (Justin Dart, Co-chair, Justice for All, 1996, address to disability organisations).

> The ADA is causing regulatory horror stories (Gingrich and Armey 1994).

As the rhetoric flows in an ideological stand-off between supporters and opponents of the ADA, debate on the ADA's achievements can become clouded. The disability community argues that the late 1990s is far too early for a full-scale review of the Act. Many of its provisions did not come into force until 1992. There is in any case little consensus on what criteria should be used to evaluate success and no full-blown evaluative data. This chapter examines the data that do exist along with examples of cases that have been through the courts, and experiences of user/survivors, advocates and attorneys, to provide a description of the first few years of progress.

Services and public places

When we think of making services, and public places, accessible, we think of things such as ramps, elevators, signers and the acceptance of guide dogs. However, the ADA – or the threat of the ADA – has been used by some mental health user/survivors and allies to challenge discrimination in areas including health care, segregation in institutions, access to programmes within prisons, 'nimby' campaigns, access to housing, and treatment by private services such as banks.

In relation to health, the court found, in *Easley* v. *Sneider* 1993, that it was unlawful for a state programme providing health maintenance to exclude those who were not 'mentally alert', because they could benefit too (Gostin, 1996). The state of Oregon, in setting its rationing criteria for health care, was required to stop ranking the quality of life of disabled people lower than that of non-disabled people (a ranking that it used to set priorities for who should and should not have access to treatments from kidney dialysis to heart surgery) (Gostin 1996).

The ADA is proving helpful in challenging the practice of segregating people in institutions. The Department of Justice states that 'integration is fundamental to the purposes of the ADA. Provision of segregated accommodations and services relegates people with disabilities to second-class status' (Rubenstein 1996). In *Helen L.* v. *DiDario* 1995, the Court held that the state of Pennsylvania violated the ADA by confining in a nursing home a plaintiff who did not require nursing home care, although by 1999 this precedent was again being challenged in the courts (cited in Bazelon Center for Mental Health Law 1997b).

The National Institute of Justice has noted that corrections establishments have to make facilities within them 'accessible' to qualified people with mental disabilities. They cannot refuse someone a status, like inmate worker – which might be helpful in obtaining work on release – on the basis of a generalised criterion such as being on psychotropic drugs (Rubin and McCampbell 1995). The FBI Law Enforcement Bulletin notes that the ADA can require accommodations in the courtroom, for example additional time to think in response to questions (Goldstein 1997).

The ADA may also be useful in challenging 'nimby' opposition to mental health facilities. Gostin (1996) notes that towns may find themselves in breach of both the Fair Housing Act 1988 and the ADA if they reject proposals for group homes for disabled people.

The threat of the ADA may be sufficient to effect a change. For example, in Berkeley, California, a consumer-run drop-in centre needed to move. The centre is used by about 80 people per day and primarily serves people from minority, especially black, communities. Many people have multiple difficulties such as extreme poverty, homelessness or criminal history. It accepts people whom many other mental health agencies either reject (many Club Houses, for example, not taking someone who is homeless or has a drug or alcohol problem), or fail to engage (for example, because a day treatment programme has rules and an air of officialdom that put people off). While this centre is highly valuable to the people who use it and is recognised as a great resource by the mental health community locally, nationally and even internationally, the people in the Berkeley neighbourhood to which it was to move in 1994 took a different view.

The local residents produced a petition, which everyone signed, opposing the drop-in. As co-ordinator Sally Zinman put it, 'we are amongst the most stereotyped in our society'. Residents lobbied everyone they could think of, arguing that their children would not be safe. The centre responded with a sophisticated political strategy, which built on connections with local decision makers forged over many years. It included asking the local Protection and Advocacy Service to write a polite letter to the council reminding them of the ADA and Fair Housing Act. The council was thus aware that its decision on the matter could not be influenced, legally, by knowing that the group had 'mental disabilities' (and indeed their own lawyers gave the same advice). The group then made a decision not to be provoked by any of the attacks on them but to respond in Martin Luther King style. If any of their members were angry in a forum discussing the issue, they left the room if necessary. Everyone stuck to this policy, and eventually the council ruled in the drop-in's favour.

They moved into the new building. Sally Zinman then encouraged people not to hang out at the front of the building. Her reasoning to other consumers was quite explicit: that her request was unfair, that if they were white and in business suits they would be accepted, but that they wanted at this point to build the local community's trust (it could hardly get much lower). They planted flowers in the front. By 1995, they won an award for beautifying the neighbourhood. There were many links with local people, they were part of the neighbourhood association that had opposed them, and the drop-in was accepted.

Before the move, in Zinman's view, there was no way in which they could have become accepted without a political battle. Mediation would not have been sufficient. Acceptance only came with familiarity and experience. Without the legal framework that required the council to take a non-discriminatory decision, they would never have had the chance to get familiar with neighbours and dissipate their fears.

This example shows how far ahead of public opinion is the law. Sally Zinman notes that people generally simply do not have a concept that it is discriminatory to throw someone out of a shop because they seem crazy, or to use language such as 'kookie' or '51 out of 50'. At this point in history, the law can be necessary, within broader strategies, to create the familiarisation that then breaks down prejudice.

Sometimes the existence of the law appears to trigger good practice in private companies. For example, a woman with severe mental health problems became very disturbed in a bank. She was yelling at the bank clerks. The bank, rather than just ejecting her – or calling the police – talked with her and agreed a solution that proved effective: she chose which bank clerk she wanted to see and made regular appointments. The local protection and advocacy agency believed that the bank's flexibility was attributable to increased disability awareness since the introduction of the ADA (Protection and Advocacy staff member, Georgia, personal communication, 1995).

Gostin (1996) concludes his review of ADA litigation with the comment that the ADA has the potential to affect 'the structure of government benefits programs, the regulation of public health and safety, and the provision of health care services in society. This is as it should be...' The Act, however, has had even more impact for users of mental health services in the sphere of employment.

Preparing employers and disabled people

Between the passage of the ADA in 1990 and the introduction of the employment provisions in 1992, a 'training the trainers' programme reached 137,000 people, including 40,000 disabled people. Mental health user/survivors were fully involved.

Technical assistance for employers and information for disabled people was made available through 10 regional Disability and Business Technical Assistance Centers and through the Job Accommodation Network, which advises approximately 81,000 inquirers per year – mainly employers. By 1993, 40% of disabled people knew of the ADA (Harris 1994), a figure that compares reasonably with public knowledge of other anti-discrimination laws. Also knowledge among employers was clearly rising (West 1996).

The technical assistance effort was not problem free. West (1996) notes that, by 1994, ADA literature was being provided free to 15,000 libraries and 7600 grocery stores. Additionally, the EEOC speakers' bureau had delivered 2300 speeches on the ADA. However, there was no co-ordination of technical assistance by numerous different agencies, a mini-industry had sprung up teaching business how not to comply with the ADA, and complaints were not dealt with promptly – the Department of Justice was turning some complaints away, and the EEOC, which had received 29,000 ADA complaints by 1994, was taking an average of 293 days to deal with each. For disabled people – including those with mental health problems, who made up 12.6% of those complaining to the EEOC – the process could be bureaucratic and time consuming.

British proposals for a Disability Rights Commission in 1998 rejected the idea of a Commission that processed every complaint, in a deliberate attempt to avoid repetition of these difficulties.

Training on specialist issues, including accommodations for people with psychiatric disabilities, was developed. Skills in training employers were 'bedded in' to mainstream organisations like Chambers of Commerce. The Washington Business Group on Health, which represents and advises Fortune 500 companies, ran a 3-year project to advise companies on employing people with psychiatric disabilities. They built a database of accommodations made in 300 companies and said:

> We have found that accommodations for people with psychiatric disabilities are fairly easy to describe. Often they are simple solutions, that employers may never have thought of, like allowing an office worker to take breaks but also take work home at weekends – for instance, if the person has a difficulty with concentration (Ann Makowski, Washington Business Group on Health, 1996).

Nonetheless, by 1996, most psychiatrically disabled people interviewed in a national study did not know about the relevance of the ADA to them, nor about the types of accommodation that could be helpful, and many employers did not know what type of accommodations would be useful for employees with mental health problems (Granger *et al.* 1996).

It is universally agreed that training, information and advice are essential to creating change; just passing a law is not enough.

Getting work

Data on changes in the employment patterns of disabled people since 1992 suggest some small room for optimism. While one study suggests that employment among disabled people (of all kinds) fell, marginally, from 33% in 1986 to 31% in 1991 (National Organization on Disability, quoted in Hudgins 1995), more recent data from the US Census Bureau showed 800,000 more seriously disabled people working in 1994 than in 1991 (*Business Week*, 10 February 1997). Longer-term monitoring is required, as this increase is partly attributable to a general growth in the US economy and may be related to specific welfare-to-work initiatives and not only to the ADA.

The main direct impact of the ADA has so far been in retaining existing staff rather than hiring new disabled people. EEOC statistics show that more complaints relate to decisions to fire an employee, or issues within the workplace such as reasonable accommodations, than to hiring. In the first 3 years of implementation of the employment provisions, only 13% of complaints concerned hiring (West 1996). For psychiatric disability specifically, this figure was only 6% (hiring and rehiring); the range of complaints is shown in Table 8.1.

Table 8.1 Complaints to the EEOC from people with psychiatric disabilities, by topic, 1993–95

	1993	1994	1995
Accommodations	308	571	734
Discipline	136	249	323
Promotion	53	80	105
Wages	36	81	94
Harassment	211	427	547
Discharge	816	1300	1457
Benefit	45	102	139
Lay-off	51	80	42
Hiring	154	150	128
Rehiring	59	66	82
Suspension	41	81	84
Other	385	675	762
Total	2295	3862	4497

Source: Unpublished data on EEOC ADA charges relating to psychiatric disability.

The low level of hiring complaints may result from the fact that discrimination in hiring is less blatant than in firing: people may not be sure why they have been turned down, and they may be disinclined to file charges against an organisation in which they have no particular investment and which has just rejected them. Psychiatrically disabled people may be less likely than others even to try applying for jobs (see Ch. 3) and, if they do, may be unlikely to decide to disclose their psychiatric history and challenge discrimination, given all the risks, unless the 'chips are down', for example if they are threatened with dismissal.

Also, accommodating existing employees may be a developmental stage for employers:

> Because of the ADA employers are now learning that they can successfully make accommodations for existing staff who develop psychiatric disabilities. The next step will be that they will extend this knowledge to hiring people: because Tom works well, they'll be prepared to employ Jane, who has the necessary skills. It's a learning process (DJ Hendricks, Job Accommodation Network, personal communication, 1996).

Of the 650 ADA cases that had been through the courts by 1995, a small number did set precedents in relation to hiring, for example through a settlement requiring ADA training for managers (Columbia Aluminium Recycling Limited, cited in Bazelon Center for Mental Health Law 1997a). Gradually, some user/survivors are beginning to think of complaining about hiring discrimination. One Virginia user told me he was taking legal advice after being offered a place on a motor industry training programme and subsequently being turned down after disclosing his psychiatric history.

The ADA may also be important in hiring in invisible ways. It is illegal under the ADA to ask questions about a person's disability – including any history of mental health treatment – on application forms or in interviews, prior to job offer. Feldblum (1996) found, from a small survey of employers, that two-thirds had made changes in application procedures as a result of the ADA, such as moving medical examinations from pre- to post-job offer; the other third already complied. Most had experienced no significant problems in complying. A minority thought that physicians had become more cautious about deeming people unfit for certain jobs, which might be beneficial for people with past mental illness, who have sometimes been excluded summarily through the medical examination process.

User/survivors may be encouraged to apply for jobs if they know that they should not be asked intrusive questions at interview. Research by Akabas and colleagues traced people who worked for the City of New York, in all types of job from street sweeper to administration, who were receiving mental health treatment. All obtained their job through open competition. Of the first 180 interviewed, about half had not disclosed their problems to their employer. Many were underemployed in relation to their educational level. Some of the supervisors who knew of the problem said they would never have found someone so qualified had it not been for the disability. For some of this group, it might have been knowledge that they had some legal protection that encouraged them to apply for these jobs in the first place (Akabas, personal communication, 1996).

One day in 1995, 200 socially disabled people packed into a church in Washington DC to learn about how to get jobs. The organisers and many of the teachers were user/survivors from the DC Consumers' League. Companies including Pizza Hut and DC Cable were present recruiting, and participants learnt about everything from training and interview support programmes to rights under the ADA and schemes run by the Social Security Administration to reduce the disincentives involved in pursuing work. A knowledge of ADA rights appeared to act as one key component in encouraging people to think that it might be possible to enter the labour force.

In Alabama, a rural state with no public transport to many areas, driving licences are essential for many jobs. User/survivors used the ADA to get the state policy on driving licence application changed. Where the forms had previously asked a general question about whether the applicant had ever suffered from mental illness, the new procedure debarred only some people with recent psychiatric problems.

Julie Clark is an attorney whose application to join the state Bar was turned down because of her prior mental health problems. The application asked whether the person had ever suffered from mental illness. She took a case under the ADA and won, being admitted to the Bar in 1996. Rubenstein (1996) describes how the practice of inquiring about a past history of mental illness in medical and legal licensing procedures is gradually being overturned by the courts. Inquiries about specific conduct are replacing the discriminatory use of 'past mental illness' as grounds for exclusion, or grounds for further investigations not applied to those with no psychiatric history. 'Additional reforms are sure to follow', Rubenstein concludes.

Staying on the job

Considerable effort has gone into defining and trying out accommodations in the workplace for psychiatrically disabled people. Examples are now available in guides (Mancuso 1993) and on the

Internet (for example, the Center for Psychiatric Rehabilitation, Boston). Similar initiatives were developed in the UK a few years later (Mind 1997b, Employers' Forum on Disability 1998).

Many people need no specific accommodations or they create their own, for example by taking a few minutes 'time out' when distressed, if the job allows, or asking for more feedback without mentioning that this is related to a 'disability' such as anxiety. A Sears Roebuck study found that fewer than 10% of employees who self-identified as disabled needed any accommodation at all to enable them to work (Blanck 1994a).

Where accommodations are needed, those for user/survivors may at first glance seem more obscure than those for other disabled people. This does not mean that they are necessarily difficult to define or to implement. For instance:

> The most common accommodation we make is to allow people with psychiatric problems, like depression, to return to work in a measured way – not to have to come back full time all at once. This works very well. Most of those people are still working today and everything is forgotten about (Dr Dan Conti, Director, Employee Assistance Program, First National Bank of Chicago, 1996).

> Simple physical changes to the workplace may be effective accommodations... For example, room dividers, partitions, or other soundproofing or visual barriers between workspaces may accommodate individuals who have disability-related limitations in concentration. Moving an individual away from noisy machinery or reducing other workplace noise that can be adjusted (for example lowering the volume or pitch of telephones)... permitting an individual to wear headphones to block out noisy distractions may also be effective (Equal Employment Opportunity Commission 1997).

> The most common accommodations we make involve changed schedules, time off for doctors' appointments or moving the person into a different role – for instance, reducing customer contact. Or sometimes they're very individual accommodations, linked to individual symptoms. We've overcome most of the barriers; it hasn't imposed major difficulties. We haven't found that people are unreliable. Since the ADA and our program to train the supervisors in all our major divisions – covering 21,000 employees – we have seen a change in the culture. Some people used to assume that if you weren't able to work 100% all the time that was a real problem. Now the managers begin by asking what the person can do. It's made savings for us – an estimated $140,000

in 1995, in benefit dollars we haven't had to pay (Bruce Flynn, Wells Fargo Bank, San Francisco, 1996).

The key to these accommodations is generally creative thinking and easy access to advice for managers, rather than cost (Feldblum 1996). A few accommodations do involve technology, for example having a computer to work at home for someone with agoraphobia, or a cueing aid that prompts a person with a cognitive impairment to follow a schedule. In the main, however, the solution is flexibility, someone to talk to, extra support or feedback.

It is important not to assume that users 'cannot cope with stress'. Mancuso has found that, for some employees, the key is to have plenty to do: they become anxious if underoccupied (Mancuso 1993).

The EEOC has specified a number of reasonable accommodations that can be adopted, depending on individual circumstances and on whether the accommodation would constitute 'undue hardship' to the particular employer. These include permitting a job coach from a mental health agency to accompany someone to work; changing workplace policies, for example allowing more breaks to obtain drinks to accommodate someone whose medication means that they need plenty of fluid; and changing managerial feedback to suit individuals, making it more frequent, or conveying it on paper or by e-mail if needed (Equal Employment Opportunity Commission 1997).

An increasing number of employers have made accommodations for disabled people generally: from 51% in 1986 to 81% in 1995 (Harris 1995). Data on the number of employers providing accommodations for psychiatric disability in particular was not available at the time of writing.

The Job Accommodation Network found that, overall, the employers it advised, on all kinds of disability, saved money by instigating accommodations. In 69% of cases, the accommodation cost less than $500; in 19% of cases, it cost nothing. Of those making an accommodation, 72% found it effective or very effective. The benefits realised included those shown in Table 8.2.

The Washington Business Group on Health found that the cost of making accommodations for people with psychiatric disabilities was lower than the cost of disability benefits. The Office of Technology Assessment found that employers were instigating accommodations for people with mental health problems in ways that

Table 8.2   Benefits reported by employers of making reasonable
accommodations for disabled people

	%*
Retaining or hiring a qualified employee	56
Eliminating the cost of training a new employee	30
Saving workers' compensation/other costs	37
Increasing workers' productivity	54
Other benefits	25

Source: JAN US Annual Report, October 1994 to September 1995 (N=683).
*Percentages do not total 100% as some respondents listed more than one benefit.

made good business sense, and in ways that suited the business
(Office of Technology Assessment 1994).

Some employers see clear advantages to employing socially
disabled people, for example:

> Dan works as a messenger at a large bank in Salem. He has a traumatic
> brain injury. He works really well as long as he has a clear routine. The
> benefit for an organisation is you don't have the constant turnover for
> positions like this, which can be a real pain... In banking in the US
> people are very aware of this trade-off. They are with the spirit of the
> ADA (Personnel Director, 1995).

Surveys of employers consistently find that they support the
ADA. A 1995 Harris poll of American corporations found the
following views on whether the ADA should be strengthened,
weakened or left alone:

Strengthen	No change	Weaken	Repeal	Don't know/refused
8%	70%	9%	3%	10%

Seventy-five per cent said that they intended to make greater
efforts to employ people with disabilities in the next 3 years. They
believed, by an 80% to 5% margin, that the opportunities of the
ADA were worth the cost of implementation. Small businesses
were as supportive of the ADA as larger ones (Harris 1995).

There is, of course, a big proviso to all this from the user's point
of view: you have to disclose that you are disabled in order to have

a right to an accommodation, something that many people, with good reason, are afraid to do (see Ch. 9 for a fuller discussion of these dilemmas). Nonetheless, for some people, knowing about the concept of reasonable accommodations can embolden them to seek them out.

In Britain, the DDA Code of Practice on Employment states that employers should do what they can to find out whether a person has a disability that places him or her at a disadvantage. For example, if someone cries at work, a manager would be expected to give the employee an opportunity to explain whether disability is an issue rather than just disciplining them for not leaving personal problems at home (Disability Discrimination Act 1995).

The British Employment Code of Practice also gives examples of reasonable adjustments that are relevant to socially disabled people – such as support at work, flexible working hours and time off for therapy or treatment.

Of course, it is not always the case that a person gets an accommodation agreed and works successfully thereafter. When things get tough, the ADA can also be useful.

Firing decisions

The EEOC had taken seven cases relating to mental disability – that is, psychiatric disability or mental impairment – by 1995, the vast majority of litigation having been brought by private individuals rather than by the EEOC. The very first ADA case taken to court by the EEOC concerned a chief executive who was diagnosed as having a brain tumour, immediately told his board and was fired. He won his case and was compensated. The board had not shown that he could not do the job, had not explored whether accommodations might help – and had broken the law (Equal Employment Opportunity Commission 1996).

In *Phelps* v. *Land Title* (1994), the appellate court upheld the lower court's finding that a person with depression had been intentionally discriminated against on the basis of disability and age. The employer agreed that the person they had replaced her with, after firing her, was less qualified for the job than she was (Bazelon Center for Mental Health Law 1997a).

Some critics of the ADA have argued that the reason for the high number of charges filed with the EEOC concerning discharge is that people who have never before mentioned that they have a disability suddenly claim stress-related disability when they are being fired or laid off as an excuse for poor performance or a routine part of any legal armoury to oppose firing decisions (see Ch. 10). While every law has its share of people who abuse it, it may equally be that people only choose to 'come out' about their impairment in a hostile work setting when the situation becomes desperate. Charges concerning psychiatric disability that result in either benefit to the employee or administrative closure ran at 18–39% in the years 1993–95 (EEOC, unpublished data); this compares favourably with outcomes of charges on race and gender discrimination. There is no evidence that people are any more likely to use 'psychiatric disability' as an excuse than other anti-discrimination law, and the idea of vast numbers of non-disabled people choosing to take on a record of psychiatric disability, with its manifold disadvantages, seems implausible.

Meeting employer criticisms of the ADA

Despite widespread support for the ADA, employers do express concerns about this law in general and about employing psychiatrically disabled people in particular. The main problems raised are reasonably straightforward to address.

Problem A. What happens when people come to work with guns?

Violence in the workplace is a growing concern for US employers. However, a look at the evidence shows that between 75% and 82% of workplace homicide is a direct result of a robber or felon (Bureau for Labor Statistics 1992, 1993, quoted in Kraus et al. 1995). Worker-on-worker homicide, committed by current or former employees, accounts for 4% of workplace homicide (Toscano and Windau 1993). A review of the literature concludes: 'efforts at curtailing robberies at the worksite would be far more effective in reducing the overall magnitude of the injury problem than trying to identify employees with a significant grudge who might choose to express their hostility at work' (Kraus et al. 1995). Professor John Monahan states that, 'the vast majority of workplace violence is in no way linked to mental disorder' (personal communication, 1996).

If employees do commit or threaten violence, they should, according to EEOC guidance, be disciplined under company policy on violence whether or not they have a 'disability'. If they commit a conduct disorder for which they are disciplined but not fired, accommodations can be explored at the same time as the disciplinary action takes place. There is, however, absolutely nothing to stop an employer firing someone who is violent: having a psychiatric disability is not seen under the ADA as any form of excuse. This applies to all conduct standards that are job-related, consistent with business necessity and applied equally to all employees.

When someone gets angry at work, there may be accommodations that can resolve the issue. The Postal Service is now developing helpful policies. For example:

> Mr X, a postal clerk, is a Vietnam veteran who has post traumatic stress disorder resulting from his wartime service. When he is given orders he sometimes gets extremely agitated or angry. He was referred for counselling to the Employee Assistance Program where he described these anxiety episodes as feeling that the walls were closing in on him and that he wanted to explode. EAP co-ordinator David Ritter explains what happened next. 'We arranged an accommodation with him such that if he felt that way he could leave the building for a short time. We gave him an "out", a safety valve. Once he had calmed down, he could come back. It has worked out very well. From having 4 or 5 anxiety attacks each month he now has them almost never. Because he knows he has an "out" his anxiety is reduced. He has never abused the arrangement. Mr X says that this system has saved his job and helped him to deal with his life' (personal communication, 1996).

Employers also have to realise that, as the EEOC eloquently puts it, 'an individual does not pose a "direct threat" simply by virtue of having a history of psychiatric disability or being treated for a psychiatric disability'. Employers are permitted to exclude individuals from work if there is evidence of specific behaviour that would pose a direct threat (to self or others), but it contravenes the ADA to assume this from a psychiatric record, or from evidence of previous suicide attempts, or from the fact that someone takes psychiatric drugs. Decisions must be based on the particular employee, in the present and future (Equal Employment Opportunity Commission 1997).

Under British anti-discrimination law, as under American, employers are in no way prevented from dismissing someone who is violent.

Problem B. What about the impact on the bottom line, and on customers, when the person is not functioning?

The law states that an employer only has to employ a person with a disability if he or she is 'qualified'. A number of court cases make it clear that if someone cannot do the essential functions of the job, the employer is within his or her rights to fire the person. For example:

> In *Larkins* v *CIBA Visions Corporation* (1994), the court stated that a worker with a panic attack disorder could not perform the essential functions of the job as a customer service representative because she could not handle customer telephone calls. The company was not required to restructure the job to include primarily non-telephone duties (Bazelon Center for Mental Health Law 1997a).

> There is no requirement to drop standards of productivity in order to employ people with disabilities (Equal Employment Opportunity Commission 1992).

As the EEOC states, 'maintaining satisfactory conduct and performance typically is not a problem for individuals with psychiatric disabilities' (Equal Employment Opportunity Commission 1997). Where it is, however, employers can take firm action to tackle it.

The same is true in Britain. Under the DDA, an employer cannot treat a disabled employee in a discriminatory way – unless it is 'justified', for example if the employee cannot fulfil the requirements of the job.

Problem C. They won't get on with co-workers

Employers often worry that if they accommodate someone by allowing them a break in the day, or an office of their own, other employees will be resentful (Feldblum 1996). These are perceived as privileges that everyone else wants too. Far from helping the disabled person, it may make their life a misery because of co-workers' envy.

Sometimes the accommodation does raise an issue of general conditions that a union or staff association may want to take up on behalf of other workers. It may be possible for everyone to work flexitime or to have improved management feedback. A labour union may sometimes oppose promoting someone on the basis of merit, under the ADA, because of a union agreement about promotion on the basis of seniority, an issue that can prompt re-negotiation to a merit-based system.

There are also suggested ways for the employer to deal with the 'envy factor'. They can inform the whole workforce about the ADA and explain that some workers may have accommodations made for invisible impairments. The Washington Business Group on Health recommends brochures, posters and outside speakers. Employee assistance staff or advocates outside the organisation can support a disabled employee in deciding whether to tell co-workers about the disability; in some cases, the advantage of reducing resentment may outweigh the fears of being treated differently, although in others the reverse may be true. NAMI's 1996 public opinion survey found that about half of respondents thought they would not tell co-workers if they had a psychiatric disability (National Alliance for the Mentally Ill 1996). The EEOC receives about 400 complaints per year of harassment against people with psychiatric histories, so people's fears of telling may be very well founded.

If the problem with co-workers is that they are having to pick up the slack from a colleague who is underperforming, this may be an 'undue hardship' under the ADA (Bazelon Center for Mental Health Law 1997a). If, however, the problem is that co-workers do not like or feel comfortable with someone just because they have a disability, that is not an undue hardship. That is prejudice and should not be tolerated any more than if white staff members object to working with African American colleagues.

In Britain, the DDA Code of Practice on Employment makes it clear that when other employees would also like the 'adjustment' that is being made for a disabled colleague, this is not likely to be significant in determining whether the adjustment is or is not 'reasonable'. The employer is likely to have to make the adjustment if co-worker envy is the only reason against it.

Problem D. It'll waste a lot of time and money in court cases

By 1995, there had been only 650 ADA court cases – about one hundredth of a per cent of all federal court cases (Gostin 1996). Far more are resolved by the EEOC or by informal means. There are no punitive damages unless wilful discrimination is proved, and none at all for state and local government. The ADA explicitly encourages the use of alternative dispute resolution rather than law alone, and mediators have been trained across the country. DREDF notes that, of 748 ADA-mediated cases examined, a settlement was reached in 400 (West 1996).

Peter Maida, a mediator with experience in the mental health field, notes that mediation can mean that mental health user/survivors set a goal for what they personally want to achieve rather than being guided by an attorney's assumption that they should go for the highest financial gain that the law allows. The negotiation process can help to correct the power imbalance that user/survivors usually experience in discussions with anyone: mediation requires that everyone is taken equally seriously. It may also enable user/survivors to learn negotiating skills that may be useful in other spheres. While some user/survivors are suspicious – will it involve negotiating below the level of their rights? Will the power really be equalised? – Maida points out that mediation has to be carried out within a legal framework so the outcome should lie clearly within the requirements of the ADA (personal communication, 1996).

The use of mediation is likely to grow. It is in the interests of government to save court costs; and employers, to save legal costs. It may often be in the interests of employees with mental health problems, for whom getting into a court case can be 'about the most stressful thing you can do' (user/survivor who had taken an ADA case to court).

In Britain, the DDA places an obligation on ACAS – the Advisory, Conciliation and Arbitration Service – to try to promote settlements of disputes without tribunal hearings.

Conclusion

One could end this chapter with a very upbeat assessment of the ADA. It is undoubtedly early days, but we have already seen some hard achievements in decisions in hiring, making accommodations and firing, as well as in non-employment fields ranging from driving licences to securing non-institutional mental health services. We might wish to conclude that the ADA really does show that the disability inclusion model is beginning to bear fruit. Employers, as the Job Accommodation Network put it, will move from making accommodations to improving their hiring practice, and as more people gain the experience, in the workplace and elsewhere, of proximity with user/survivors, old myths and stereotypes will gradually fade. The ADA, together with related laws – such as the Fair Housing Act 1988 and Individuals with Disabilities in Education Act 1975 – will create the conditions for familiarity with user/survivors, which will have a cumulative effect on attitudes and behaviour in ways that could never be achieved by public education alone. Ultimately all disabled people, including those who are socially disabled, will be able to move into mainstream life.

However, this optimistic version of events fails to take into account some rather more fundamental problems with the ADA, which may limit, although not destroy, its potential, as we shall see in the next chapter.

CHAPTER 9

The Limits of the Law

For all the impressive ADA implementation activity (see Ch. 8), there are certain types of discrimination, identified in Chapter 3, that were not even touched by the ADA in its first years.

Parental rights

Chapter 3 noted that the taboo on parenting by people with mental health problems reveals deep-rooted discrimination. Has the ADA helped?

Five years after the ADA's introduction, legal challenges to parental rights terminations under the ADA had been 'universally unsuccessful' (*Disability Compliance Bulletin* 1996). When the ADA was passed, little was done to 'even consider... the use of psychiatric categories to make decisions about parental rights' (Rubenstein 1996). Specific parental rights law – which can be highly discriminatory in its application – often takes precedence over disability discrimination law. The *Disability Compliance Bulletin* recommended renewed legal challenges under the ADA in order to set new precedents.

In some US states parental rights have been eroded. Limits have been placed on the length of time that children can stay in foster care before parental rights are terminated: in Minneapolis, a 12-month limit was introduced in the mid-1990s. The already distant possibility that people with mental health problems could be supported to raise children may recede further.

The ADA did not originally clearly prohibit genetic discrimination. By 1990, 6% of Fortune 500 companies had already carried out genetic testing of employees, and a 1989 survey suggested that 15% of companies planned to do so (Gostin 1993). The ADA protected people who had a current disability or a history of disability – but not explicitly those with a possible future disability, who might be refused work or insurance as a result. This omission was later addressed by advocacy organisations pushing for new legislation and by EEOC guidance.

Britain's DDA does not cover genetic discrimination: it only covers progressive conditions once they have become disabling.

Non-discrimination in treatment: the right to access and the right to say no

At present, mental health law, permitting involuntary detention and treatment, takes priority over anti-discrimination law, even though anti-discrimination principles might throw into question the entire basis of mental health law (as was discussed in Ch. 6).

When it comes to having access to mental health treatment, on a non-discriminatory basis, the ADA has not helped much either. The ADA does make clear that an employer can adopt health insurance that excludes people with pre-existing conditions, as long as this is not done as a subterfuge to evade the purposes of the ADA. However, despite considerable lobbying to get parity in health insurance accepted by the EEOC as an aspect of non-discrimination in employment, the EEOC ruled the other way. Their argument was that an insurance policy would be discriminatory if it were less favourable to all people with a disability or to a particular category of disability (such as blindness) but not if it were less favourable to a group of disabilities, for example 'mental illness'. No one in the disability community could see the logic of this argument – Feldblum (1996) calling it 'more a prudent approach to the political winds than a persuasive legal document' – but the EEOC appeared to take the view that Congress was the place to address parity in health insurance, which they did in 1996 (see Ch. 4).

Anti-discrimination law itself does not come in and revolutionise existing law and procedure. Legal change is a dynamic process in which cases under anti-discrimination law can establish new precedents but can equally be trumped by other laws framed in more discriminatory paradigms.

In Britain, the DDA regulations permit less favourable occupational pension benefits – including those for accident, death or invalidity – where actuarial evidence shows that the cost for this employee will be substantially greater than that for other employees. The disabled employee may still have to pay the same contri-

bution as other employees, even if he or she is not entitled to the
same rate of benefits (Disability Discrimination Act 1995).

Access to services and public accommodations

The ADA has also not prevented new, discriminatory measures
being introduced.

When people want to buy a gun, they are now, in many US states,
supposed to be checked out for history of psychiatric admission. This
was not a measure that mental health users actively opposed: the
right of 'crazy' people to bear arms did not seem the most politically
winnable proposition (although John Monahan did write one article
for the *Boston Globe* explaining that these exemptions would fail to
address America's violent crime problem and were discriminatory).
Every time the National Rifle Association (NRA) tries to reassure
people about the safety of gun ownership, and every time newspapers carry debates on gun control, a clause appears explaining that
felons and ex-psychiatric patients are ineligible. For example:

> The NRA says a law passed in Florida in 1987 has been the model for
> right-to-carry laws passed by other states. The Florida law allows adults
> who do not have criminal records or a history of mental illness or
> alcohol abuse and who have been trained in safe firearm use to carry
> concealed firearms (*Washington Times*, 1 January 1996).

This entrenches the notion that everyone who has been in a psychiatric hospital is likely to be violent. Many of the 28 states allowing
concealed handguns by 1996 modelled their law on Florida's.

For some in the mental health community, the law's limitations
mean that the ADA is not necessarily the highest priority – even if
their whole mission is to combat discrimination. One academic
concerned about the erosion of health care entitlement told me that
the ADA was marginal to many disabled people's lives.

Employment

In the sphere of employment, problems can still arise because the
ADA is not a pure 'disability rights' law: it also contains remnants
of the other models discussed in Chapters 4–7, which can at times
undermine its anti-discriminatory intent.

The moral taint of psychiatric disability

Some groups of people are explicitly excluded from the ADA. In some cases, this is simply a question of keeping up with current thinking on what is and is not an impairment: homosexuality has not been classified as a mental disorder since 1973 and is therefore not covered. Other exclusions are more controversial, for example the current use of illegal drugs (although people who are in or have been through rehabilitation are covered, as are those with current alcoholism), kleptomania, pyromania, compulsive gambling and all kinds of sexual behaviour disorder not resulting from physical impairments (for example, transsexualism, exhibitionism, voyeurism and paedophilia).

Rubenstein has argued that this 'combination of moral confusion and 19th century medicine' renders the ADA imperfect (Rubenstein 1993). Bob Burgdorf, one of the originators of the ADA, stated that the exclusion of certain disabilities was 'a low moment in American politics' (Burgdorf, personal communication, 1996). There is undoubtedly room for discussion about whether all these categories should be thought of as psychiatric disorders. Nevertheless, if these states are in the DSM, people can face employment discrimination because they are assumed to be 'sick' or 'crazy' (for example, if they have a history of one of these conditions) when they may be fully able to do the job.

Morally based exclusions mean that people with drug addiction can be randomly tested and fired from jobs even when their addiction has no bearing on performance (as discussed in Ch. 2). Those with both drug and mental health problems could, in theory, make an ADA claim about discrimination based on their mental illness. It is unlikely, however, that they would. They are not inclined to trust that a law explicitly excluding them on one count will treat them fairly on another.

In Britain, the DDA followed the American example by creating specific exclusions: the tendency to set fires, steal, physically or sexually abuse other persons; exhibitionism; voyeurism; and – going beyond the American exclusions – addiction/dependency on alcohol or any non-prescribed substance. This means that there is no protection from discrimination even for people with past alcohol or drug problems (unless they have a secondary impairment, such as liver damage, consequent on the addiction).

Paternalism and control

The ADA is widely perceived, in many ways correctly, as a law that breaks from the tradition of treating disabled people with a mixture of paternalism and control, but the remnants of older ideas remain.

First, under the ADA, an employer may have the right not to hire someone who may pose a threat to *him or herself*. Rubenstein (1993) notes that the disability movement's charges of paternalism have not been laid to rest by EEOC assurances that 'direct threat' must be based on individualised assessment, supported by reasonable medical judgement, using the most current medical knowledge and/or the best available objective evidence. Individualised assessments could still mean someone being refused a job because they have once before had difficulty under stress – even if a repeat experience would risk neither work performance nor anyone else's safety. In any event, 'the business of the employer is to get the job done and allow employees to watch out for themselves', as Rubenstein puts it.

Given employers' vested interests in keeping health insurance costs down, they could try to manage the financial risk by using this provision to keep people out of the workforce who may become sick. From the point of view of user/survivors, this amounts to being kept out of society supposedly 'for their own good' all over again.

The second problem concerns power and control. In particular, who decides what is a reasonable accommodation in the workplace? Under the ADA it is up to the employee to seek an accommodation, but his or her views can ultimately be overruled by the employer, for example if the employer can suggest an effective and less expensive alternative. The aim, which is often realised, is to reach an amicable agreement (Mancuso 1993).

Some employers have thought it appropriate to require someone to take medication – or even to monitor whether they take it – as part of this 'accommodation'. All the organisations advising employers with whom I spoke had come across employers wanting to take, or taking, this approach. An EEOC spokesperson told me 'it comes up all the time'. One employer remarked:

> I think the ADA could be amended so that a person could have to be in treatment, if they want to have the accommodation. That's give and take, the company is putting itself out for them, and they're making their effort; and it's therapeutic.

For the first few years of ADA implementation, groups like the Washington Business Group on Health advised employers, correctly, that there had been no EEOC ruling on this issue, which rather implied that employers were free to require employees to take medication. Users objected: 'it doesn't make any difference if you get the work done by taking Prozac or standing on your head. The thing that matters is the work' (employee, 1996), and user/ survivors Howie the Harp and Judi Chamberlin emphasised that accommodations must be voluntary. User/survivors were, not unreasonably, nervous that the ADA might lead to an intrusion of psychiatric control into the workplace. This danger may be especially acute when – as in many workplaces – the information most available is framed in terms of the 'brain disease' model, emphasising that people can live productive lives with the right medication rather than through a whole variety of strategies that must remain within users' control.

In 1997, the EEOC Guidance clarified the position, in user/ survivors' favour: 'medication monitoring is not a reasonable accommodation'. In addition, if a person is engaging in 'misconduct' apparently as a result of not taking medication, 'the employer should focus on the employee's conduct and explain to the employee the consequences of continued misconduct in terms of uniform disciplinary procedures. It is the employee's responsibility to decide about medication and to consider the consequences of not taking medication' (Equal Employment Opportunity Commission 1997). Compliance with this guidance requires careful monitoring.

The issue of psychiatric control also comes up in jails. A US National Institute of Justice briefing states that it may be acceptable under the ADA to require that someone takes medication in order for them to participate in a particular programme (Rubin and McCampbell 1995). Such attempts to control people's medication as part of giving *them* greater rights and access would be virtually unthinkable in the field of physical illness.

In Britain, under the DDA, the Code of Practice states that if an employee refuses to follow occupational medical advice provided on behalf of the employer about methods of working or *managing his condition at work* (my italics), and the condition deteriorates, the employer may subsequently be justified in not making further adjustments (which might presumably include those which the user believes helpful).

American dreams, American fantasies

> I have a dream. It is a dream deeply rooted in the American dream, that one day this nation will rise up and live out the true meaning of its creed – we hold these truths to be self-evident, that all men are created equal (Martin Luther King, March on Washington, 1963).

In 1996, Cornell West noted that, since this speech, a quarter of African Americans had joined the middle classes and become materially better off, while fully a third were worse off than before (paper presented in Washington DC, 1996). The civil rights movement had sparked major social change and ended outright exclusion from specific industries, but its laws had not redressed entrenched imbalances of power, wealth and status (West and Gates 1996). As West (1994) illustrates: 'After the ninth [New York] taxi refused me my blood began to boil. The tenth taxi refused me and stopped for a kind, well-dressed, smiling female fellow citizen of European descent.'

In the 1990s, disability activists and supportive politicians spoke as powerfully of the American dream:

> With the enactment of this landmark civil rights law... our people began coming together to ensure equal access to the American dream (President Bill Clinton, 1995).

The ADA may contain within it the seeds of a pattern of employment opportunity similar to that of earlier Civil Rights laws: while a group of more privileged disabled people benefit, for others life stays the same or even gets worse.

In the first few years of ADA implementation, the law appeared to bring most benefit to those who already had certain advantages. It benefited those already in work (as we saw in Ch. 8), but the majority of people with long-term mental health problems were not in work. It benefited white, educated people. Blanck (1994b) found that, from the 1980s, the income of white disabled people began to rise but that people of colour fared less well. Burkhauser and Daly (1996) found that, in the late 1980s, black disabled men had incomes only 25% of the level for non-black disabled men; the disparity was only slightly less severe between black and non-black women. Disabled men with poor education had an income of 28% the level of those with at least a high-school education. The authors argue that those with the negotiating power to benefit from the ADA will continue to be 'disproportionately white, male, highly educated professionals and managers'.

Many people with long-term mental health problems do not have educational qualifications, often because their difficulties emerge in adolescence. One survey of users in Southern Texas found that 85%, over double the rate for the local population generally, did not have a high-school diploma (Carlos Perez, Executive Director, Ahead-Adelante, personal communication, 1996). People developing mental health problems who are already brain researchers, senior advisors to politicians, national journalists, professors of psychiatry and the like (all actual examples of roles occupied by people who are open about having serious mental health problems) will find it easier to find and keep work than those competing for jobs in fast food chains:

> I had a job as a researcher on tax issues. My boss was angry with me because I was late in the mornings. And I was not a normal employee generally – but I was a very good researcher. So I pointed out how valuable I was. He didn't say anything – he looked a bit shocked, maybe impressed by my nerve. A little later he gave me a raise (man, Austin, Texas, 1996).

This approach is less likely to be effective in an ordinary minimum wage job, where there may be hundreds of people – waiting in the wings – ready to replace the person who arrives late for work. Many employers are anyway anxious about placing people with mental health problems in customer service roles: the shift from manufacturing to service industries in many localities has not aided user/survivors' competitive position.

The law appears to benefit those perceived to have less severe problems. Employers cite greater success in accommodating people with relatively mild depression, anxiety, post-traumatic stress disorder and perhaps bipolar disorder. 'Psychotic disorders are more of a challenge. That is much more difficult', as one Employee Assistance Programme staff member put it to me. Research suggests that a particular diagnosis is not a reliable predictor of work performance (Anthony et al. 1995). Experience from mental health employment programmes suggests considerable success in employing people with diagnoses of schizophrenia and other psychotic problems, both in supported and unsupported employment (Sherman and Porter 1991, Perkins et al. 1997), but employers do not know of this research. Also some people, with a variety of diagnoses, do have difficulty working without considerable support – in some cases more support than an employer can offer without 'undue hardship'. As a result:

> The ADA has had most impact on those who are marginally disabled – people whose disability really does not affect their performance (EAP Director 1996).

> The ADA is pretty irrelevant to us. A lot of the people we see won't find jobs anyway (consumer at a consumer-run drop-in centre 1995).

There are a number of possible methods whereby this problem could be tackled: giving employers summaries of research and practice information so that they do not make assumptions about which types of mental health problem they can or cannot accommodate; making government, rather than employers, primarily responsible for funding reasonable accommodations, thereby shifting public policy from 'the stick of ADA mandates to the carrot of accommodation tax credits' (Burkhauser and Daly 1996); promoting a greater use of existing tax breaks for ADA compliance for psychiatric disability (Mancuso 1993); and increasing the use of supported employment, which can enable employers to take on disabled staff with less risk – and with support for line managers (as will be discussed in Ch. 12).

The law may benefit people at moments of economic upturn – with uncertain consequences on the downturn. Berkowitz (1996) has argued that Congress accepted the proposal for the ADA during the 1980s 'boom', when disabled people's productive labour was wanted, but 'by the time the ADA was passed and put into operation... the boom was over and the economy had begun to deteriorate'. This added fuel to the increasing number of people claiming disability benefits. By 1997, disabled people who were *not* working were beginning to enter the workforce (see Ch. 8), although whether they would continue to increase their hold in the labour market, or be laid off again as 'marginal labour' at the next downturn, remained to be seen.

The operation of meritocracy is further distorted by social security disincentives. Both the Office of Technology Assessment (1994) and Blanck (1994b) found disincentives to be severe, especially because the loss of benefits may bring with it an end to Medicaid entitlement:

I just couldn't afford to lose the Medicaid, because of all the drugs I am on. It would have cost me hundreds of dollars a month – and the pay wasn't good enough (user/survivor, California, 1996).

There are at least 50 definitions of disability in use in federal policy alone. This can mean that one could be 'disabled' under the ADA (but not 'qualified' for the job) but still not 'disabled' enough to get disability benefits. Equally, one might undermine a case for workers' compensation by successfully arguing, under the ADA, that being 'disabled' did not mean that one could not work, whereas for workers' compensation, one must show an inability to work in order to count as 'disabled'.

A number of solutions have been proposed and in some cases piloted. The National Academy of Social Insurance (1996) suggested improved buy-ins to Medicaid and Medicare, and a refundable tax credit to employees that subsidises low wages. In a policy climate of state-level decision making within tight spending constraints, however, the chances of generalised solutions that integrate disability, health and employment policy in such a way as to ease people's transition into work seem slightly remote.

Finally, the ADA itself contains some double-binds, which can limit its potential to mitigate the impact of exclusion. There can be a very narrow window between showing that you do indeed have a disability and showing that it is not so disabling as to make you 'unqualified' for a job:

> In *Thompson* v. *City of Arlington* 1994 the Court found that a woman with depression was not a person with a 'disability' because she was asserting that she could return to her job as a police officer after medical leave (Bazelon Center for Mental Health Law 1997a).

Had this woman been unable to return to her job, she might well not have been seen as 'qualified'. At worst, if one is 'qualified', one is not 'disabled' and vice versa.

Working is considered to be a major life activity under the ADA, and sometimes the courts expect someone to be 'substantially limited' across a whole range of jobs in order to demonstrate he or she is 'disabled' (even though EEOC Guidance states that the courts should examine other major life activities before 'working'). This makes demonstrating that one is 'disabled' quite a challenge. For example:

In *Muller* v. *Automobile Club of Southern California* 1995, an insurance company claims adjuster who developed post-traumatic stress disorder after being threatened by a customer was found by the court to be capable of doing similar work for other employers. Thus, the court held, she was not a person with a disability (Bazelon Center for Mental Health Law 1997a).

Some of these problems could be reduced if the law used a wider definition of 'disability' to demonstrate outright discrimination than to stake a claim to accommodations. It seems fair to have to demonstrate substantial limitation in major life activities to qualify for accommodations because they may pose costs for the employer. A broad 'continuum' model, in which we all experience some level of mental distress, will not wash with employers (nor with the public; see Ch. 5): employers reasonably want to distinguish between the person who does experience disabling concentration problems, and needs a private room to work, and the person who dislikes noise and simply wants their own room.

But if one is refused a job because of a history of psychiatric treatment that did not, at the time, substantially limit major life activities and was not perceived by the employer to have done so – one has still not got the job. Why should there be no grounds for challenge? Using the same definition in both cases leads to the presumption in law that it is acceptable to refuse someone a job because you think that they are slightly disabled but not if you think they are substantially so. It suggests that the idea, from the social model, that prejudice can be disabling has not quite been embraced. The ADA does outlaw discrimination against people only 'regarded as' disabled, but what they are 'regarded as' having has to be an impairment that is substantially limiting. This is a social model still tinged with older ideas. In 1998, a proposal to learn from this experience in Britain, by outlawing discrimination on the basis of a wide definition of disability, but using a much narrower definition for entitlement to reasonable adjustments, was discussed but rejected because it was thought it might open the floodgates and provoke public resistance. It was thus likely to remain quite legal to refuse someone a job because of a history of minor anxiety.

A further problem is the complexity of many ADA mental health cases. There can be differences of view about performance, which can be harder to measure than in cases of physical impairment. It is a matter of judgement whether someone's approach with customers is acceptable or not and therefore whether they are facing discrimination. Some attorneys note that, faced with such differences of opinion, it is easy for judges to be swayed by the employer because the subject of mental illness 'touches such a deep vein of prejudice'. Even where the EEOC has provided guidance based on anti-discriminatory principles, the courts may revert to entrenched ideas in their judgements.

For people who are disabled – but not too disabled – and who have skills, and social advantages, the ADA could bring real social participation of a kind never achieved before. For those whose impairments mean they need more support, or those who are unskilled or lacking in social resources, the picture could be significantly gloomier.

The challenge is to integrate anti-discrimination law with policy in other areas – employment, social security and housing to name but a few – and to fuse rights-based thinking with attention to the social safety net, which provides a bedrock of security from which to move into new opportunities. Just shaking people free of the 'dependency culture' and giving them an anti-discriminatory law is unlikely to transform the position of user/survivors as a whole.

In the UK, there have been more robust national entitlements to benefit than in the US – but benefit disincentives to work are nonetheless considerable (Bray 1998). There is less experience of supported employment (Pozner *et al.* 1996), there are specific geographical areas with few or no available jobs (Donnison 1998), and the DDA has in-built contradictions at least as restrictive as the ADA.

Undermined by discrimination?

When attorney Steve Schwartz set up a project in Massachusetts specifically to represent people with severe mental health problems in challenging discrimination, he found that, after years of being institutionalised or otherwise depowered, many did not see discrimination when it was staring them in the face. Mental health professionals too may come to see discrimination against their clients as a normal part of life. It becomes almost invisible, and combating it is not a consideration. Among professionals who, in 1996, told me that they had not realised that the ADA even applied to people with mental health problems, were a director of social work in a state mental hospital and a nationally eminent psychiatrist.

If user/survivors want to seek a 'reasonable accommodation' or file a complaint about discrimination, they have to disclose. A study of Sears Roebuck notes that no database had been set up on psychiatric, as opposed to other, disabilities for data collection purposes because people with psychiatric disabilities preferred not to disclose (Blanck 1994a). Members of a Washington user group told me that they would all prefer not to disclose at work. For some user/survivors, the fear of disclosure makes the ADA irrelevant.

Some people have disclosed and been met with suspicion, their every action being interpreted as a possible symptom, or with harsher treatment. Some report being passed over for promotion – 'she wouldn't be able to handle the stress' – or laid off first when redundancies occur. Others have more positive experiences:

> Disclosing my manic depressive illness was freeing. I am at peace with myself. I have not suffered because of my disclosure. I may in the future – telling is a risky business. My story is a success story. Others are not so fortunate (La Polla 1995).

Fisher (1995) advises discussing disclosure with peers – other users – and then, if one decides to go ahead, picking someone one can trust. There is a catch-22 at play here, in that discrimination will probably only be eroded as people are more open, but discrimination stops people from being open and from availing themselves of the very law designed to stop discrimination.

In some cases, the courts have taken a limited view of the expectations placed on employers when people do not fully disclose or when they are not totally explicit about asking for an accommodation. In *Taylor* v. *the Principal Financial Group* (1996), Mr Taylor informed his employer that he had been diagnosed with bipolar disorder and asked his boss to speak with the company doctors and then schedule another meeting. The boss asked if he was 'all right', to which the employee said, 'Yeah, I guess'. On this basis, the court decided that Mr Taylor had not requested a reasonable accommodation, and the employer was not obliged to identify the need for one (Bazelon Center for Mental Health Law 1997a).

Finally, taking a case to court as a user/survivor can mean that one's psychiatric history is dragged through the courts, rather as a woman's sexual history has often been in rape cases. One user/survivor – who won her case to get meetings rescheduled as her medication regime made an 8 am start unmanageable – told me:

It was a trauma to go through the court case. Having my psychiatrist saying my diagnosis in front of people I didn't know was a real tearful moment, and talking of the deep and dark side of my symptoms. My family members said, why does it have to be you doing this? Sometimes I felt suicidal. Immediately after I'd won I felt, why did I do this? Later, once I had some distance, I was glad I'd done it (user/survivor, Texas, 1996).

The fear of such experiences stops many people availing themselves of the ADA at all.

Anti-discrimination law in other countries

It may reasonably be asked whether any countries other than the US have resolved the contradictions and pitfalls that appear evident in the early implementation of the ADA.

Britain

The UK clearly lags behind the US. In 1978 – 5 years after the passage of America's Rehabilitation Act (see Ch. 8) – the Labour Secretary of State for Employment said he doubted that there was sufficient discrimination on mental health grounds to warrant new law, despite a dossier of cases delivered to him by Mind. In 1990, the Conservative Employment Secretary frankly admitted to a House of Commons Employment Committee that the government approached the matter of disability discrimination law 'with a predisposition that a convincing case has not been made out' (Bynoe *et al.* 1991).

It was only when a later Minister, Nicholas Scott, was shamed by his own daughter – a disability organisation lobbyist – for blocking a civil rights Bill by planting questions to get it 'talked out' that the government began to take note of the disability movement and brought in the (limited) Disability Discrimination Act 1995.

This DDA adopted a more medical than social model of disability (Gooding 1996). A user of mental health services could be forgiven for assuming that she or he is included only reluctantly:

> The Act states that it *does not* [my italics] include any impairment resulting from or consisting of a mental illness, unless that illness is a clinically well-recognised illness (Disability Discrimination Act 1995).

This contrasts markedly with the ADA's much broader coverage of people 'substantially impaired' in everyday activities and with the positive tone of the American EEOC Guidance, which states that Congress intended the ADA to cover discrimination against people with psychiatric disability, and the fears, myths and stereotypes upon which it is based (Equal Employment Opportunity Commission 1997). It may be that the British government feared criticism if it included psychiatric disability too positively, given attacks on the ADA for its coverage of mental illness and addiction (as we shall see in Ch. 10).

The illustrative list of impairments in 'normal day to day activities', used to define disability, include memory and the ability to concentrate or understand – but not interaction with others, as under the ADA. The British list is generally more relevant to people with learning disabilities than mental health problems.

The DDA did not cover those 'regarded as' disabled at all: it applied only to those who are or have been 'disabled' for 12 months or more – or who expected to be. Someone refused a job because of past treatment for 1 or 11 months of depression was not covered.

Unlike the ADA, the DDA did not prohibit medical examinations before job offer, although it is 'probably unlawful' to single out disabled candidates and not others for medical checks (Disability Discrimination Act 1995). Neither did it outlaw questions about disability on application forms and at interview, although the Code of Practice does state that the questions should not be used to discriminate. Nevertheless, questions potentially asked only of those with psychiatric histories, such as whether someone can handle stress, may significantly ease the process of invisible discrimination.

The DDA did not require freedom from discrimination in education. The original law had no enforcement body, although this was quickly addressed by the incoming Labour government in the late 1990s. There was no systematic implementation plan equivalent to the American cascade training model (see Ch. 8).

So flawed did the British disability movement feel this law to be that, whereas American disability activists regularly celebrate the birthday of the ADA, British activists commemorated the first anniversary of the DDA by staging a Westminster demonstration against it.

In Northern Ireland, a Fair Employment Commission, with a remit to tackle religious discrimination, has far sharper teeth, including the monitoring of workforce composition.

The 1997 Labour government, with a manifesto commitment to comprehensive and enforceable civil rights, set up a Ministerial Task Force to create improvements.

European and global approaches

In 1995, non-governmental organisations, in coalition for the European Day of Disabled Persons, published a report on the pervasive discrimination faced by Europe's 37 million disabled citizens. It noted that the European Union's (EU's) own employment policy condoned discrimination against qualified disabled applicants, who had to rely on the goodwill of individual managers to secure reasonable accommodations. It stated that the EU's much-heralded free movement of citizens and labour did not apply to many disabled people. A 1989 case in the European Court of Justice ruled that a German national employed in a supported setting in Holland was not a 'Community worker' and therefore not entitled to a residence permit and other associated benefits under Community law (European Day of Disabled Persons 1995).

In 1996, the European Commission adopted a 'communication' on equal opportunities for disabled people. It did not require specific action on the part of member countries – given commitment to the principle of 'subsidiarity' or individual country control – but encouraged member states to 'mainstream' disabled people rather than concentrate on segregated facilities. It promoted the UN Standard Rules on the Equalisation of Opportunity for Disabled People (United Nations 1993), the most far-reaching official global document to date on disability rights. The Rules assert that 'States have a responsibility to create the legal basis for measures to achieve the objectives of full participation and equality for persons with disabilities' (Rule 15); that 'any discriminatory provision against persons with disabilities must be eliminated' – with sanctions for violations (Rule 15(2)); and that states should involve disabled people's organisations in determining policy (Rule 18). In addition, the UN Committee on Economic, Social and Cultural Rights (1994) explicitly states that the denial of 'reasonable accommodation' amounts to prohibited discrimination (United Nations 1994). The Standard Rules have been subject to international monitoring: each UN country is obliged to examine how they are being applied across different areas of government activity.

Most earlier international human rights documents did not mention disability at all, and those on mental health were based on a blend of anti-discrimination principles and paternalism. The UN Resolution on the Protection of Persons with Mental Illness and the Improvement of Mental Health Care, while making mention of anti-discrimination, approves of states administering involuntary treatment to people who 'unreasonably' withhold consent 'having regard to the patient's own safety or the safety of others'; accepts physical constraint and seclusion if they are conducted according to the rules of the facility (apparently whatever these rules may be) and if it is seen (presumably by professionals) as the only means available of preventing imminent harm; and approves involuntary detention where not to do so is likely to lead to serious deterioration in the patient's condition (United Nations 1992).

In 1997, a provision to counter disability discrimination was for the first time written into the Treaty establishing the European Community. It was not especially strongly worded. The European Commission 'may take appropriate action' to combat discrimination on grounds including disability. In addition, under a 'declaration', Community institutions shall, when they draw up measures in relation to harmonisation of the single market, 'take account of the needs of persons with a disability' (appended to Article 100A).

At the same time, a European Committee on Human Rights and Psychiatry in 1998 examined options for legal change that included the possibility of compulsory treatment in the community. International and European disability rights developments could be counteracted by the global spread of interest in laws allowing compulsion in wider circumstances.

These European and global anti-discrimination initiatives are more recent than the ADA and less tested. European measures may have the potential to integrate a long-standing commitment to a social safety net with a new commitment to civil rights, thereby partly avoiding the American problem of providing American dream opportunities for some while others remain severely excluded. The European Commission's 'communication' notes problems of exclusion in education, work, mobility/access, housing *and welfare systems* (my italics). Conversely, Europe may use the opportunity of civil rights to reduce welfare 'dependency' without securing full social inclusion, perhaps especially in Britain given its 'special relationship' with the US (see Ch. 2).

While a number of individual countries within and outside Europe have introduced disability discrimination laws (for example, Australia), general human rights protections covering disability (for instance, Canada) or constitutional amendments covering disability discrimination (for example, Germany), it remains the case that 'in no other country [than the US] has legislative protection from the unfair discrimination faced by disabled people been so comprehensively and meticulously formulated' (Bynoe *et al.* 1991). The People's Republic of China Protection of the Disabled Law (1990) is the one 'outlier' aiming to enhance social, rather than individual, rights and responsibilities – disabled people being expected 'in the spirit of optimistic progress to have self-respect and self-belief, and strengthen themselves and support themselves, in order to contribute to the construction of socialism' (Article 10) – in return for which there are employment quotas. However, the law also supports eugenics. 'Idiots breed idiots' as Premier Li Peng put it when China passed a eugenics law in 1995 (quoted in *Independent*, 30 August 1997).

Conclusion

Although the ADA is a powerful tool to tackle discrimination, it does have its limitations. Some – such as the fact that many people do not dare avail themselves of it for fear of the very discrimination it is designed to challenge – could diminish in time, albeit slowly. Some are being stripped away in a dynamic process of legal interpretation and enforcement. The EEOC, for example, has responded to identified weaknesses in the law, such as the practice among some employers of insisting that someone takes medication as part of a 'reasonable accommodation'. Not all weaknesses have, however, been addressed – and not in ways that are binding.

Other problems are more fundamental: the fact that the ADA has been so easily overridden by other law, such as parental rights law; the fact that the law and its interpretation contain remnants of models that are not about disability rights but instead about paternalism and control; and the fact that the definitions – especially the single definition of disability used both to qualify for accommodations and to be free of outright discrimination – can make it hard to demonstrate that one is both 'disabled' and 'qualified'.

Even where the EEOC has promoted a more fully rights-based approach, its views have often not been echoed by actual decisions in the courts, which have sometimes reverted to old prejudices.

As long as the mix of court decisions continues to contain so many 'double-bind' cases, in which being seen as 'disabled' means you are not seen as 'qualified' and vice versa, and as long as some decisions imply that employees should 'fit in' rather than expecting employers to think creatively about accommodations, there will continue to be a strong view among many user/survivors that it is not worth disclosing at work if one can avoid it.

Lessons from the black civil rights movement suggest that the disability civil rights model itself needs to be integrated with an attention to the social safety net and interlocking areas of public policy including housing, social security and criminal justice. In addition, discrimination has to be addressed as it occurs on the cross-cutting grounds of employment status, gender, race and other factors. Both Blanck (1994b) and the Office of Technology Assessment (1994) conclude that the law itself is not sufficient to reduce the exclusion of either people with severe disabilities or those facing discrimination on multiple grounds.

While many countries are developing anti-discrimination laws, none has solved the problems evident in the ADA, although in some cases their attempts to integrate individual rights with social responsibilities may ultimately give them a greater potential to reduce social exclusion.

Critical legal studies theory would say that it is no surprise that a civil rights law like the ADA has such drawbacks since the drafting and implementation of any law is part of social discourse. It is not some neutral arbiter outside the social process: it is framed and interpreted within a context of (often reactionary) precedent, meaning that even the most progressive law gets bogged down and contradicted by other legal interpretation. There are essentially two versions of this theory: one concluding that law is therefore not a motor for social change (see, for example, Olsen 1991), the other saying that it is part of a dynamic for change, along with other aspects of public discourse and political action (see, for example, Schneider 1991).

The analysis of the ADA, in this chapter and the last, suggests that it is already having some effects on 'discourse', and on behaviour in the workplace, housing zoning decisions and people's confidence to come out, all of which are contradicted by other forces tending towards continuing or even increased discrimination. This fits the second version of critical legal studies thinking. The law alone will not change the world – but it can play its part within a broader, dynamic process.

Influencing law – taking cases, filing amicus briefs, making new legal arguments – is critical to overcoming discrimination, as are practice guidance, technical assistance, training and advice, which enable everyone from judges to employers to put law into practice. The lawyers, survivor organisations, protection and advocacy agencies, academics and policy makers who have influenced how the ADA is interpreted and used in relation to people with mental health problems have made history. Yet law alone will not create the level of historical change required.

CHAPTER 10

Public Debate, Political Action

If law alone will not usher in social inclusion, we need to understand the context in which law is framed, passed and interpreted, in order to identify methods of intervening in these social and cultural arenas.

Justin Dart, who as a Republican and a leader of disabled people played a key role in building bipartisan alliances and support for the ADA, said:

> I had always imagined the moment when the ADA would be signed into law. We would be there on the White House lawn, the band would play and it would be a triumphant moment, like at the end of the movies. When the day came I was sitting next to the President as he signed it, and suddenly I wondered why I felt oppressed. I felt an enormous weight of responsibility. We'd promised people around the world that we were going to make this thing successful. How long would it be before somebody would try it again? Then I realized this was not an end but a beginning. There was so much more to do. I cancelled the week's holiday I had planned and got back to work (Justin Dart, personal communication, 1995).

Shapiro has argued that the ADA is a law that is trying to lead, rather than follow, public opinion – more so, in his view, than the civil rights laws of the 1960s (Shapiro 1993). The black civil rights leaders did lead, however, even when they were expected by politicians to wait. When the state of Arkansas (illegally) refused to let black children into Little Rock High, President Eisenhower, as a justification for initially doing nothing, used the argument that change could not happen faster than the public would accept. His hand was forced by Arkansas' decision to bring in troops to keep the black students out (at which point he ordered federal troops in – and the rest is history). When, in the 1960s, Martin Luther King was criticised by moderate clergy for wanting too much change too fast, he wrote the famous letter from the Birmingham jail:

> For years now I have heard the word 'wait'. It rings in the ear of every negro with a piercing familiarity. This 'wait!' has almost always meant 'never!'... We have waited for more than 340 years for our constitutional and God-given rights... There comes a time when the cup of endurance runneth over (quoted in Southern Poverty Law Center 1989).

The black civil rights movement did not wait for public opinion.

In the current state of our democracy, public opinion is often poorly informed. In 1996, a *Washington Post* survey found that 40% of those surveyed did not know that the Republicans controlled both the Senate and House of Representatives (*Washington Post*, 29 January 1996). Hume (1995) points out that 60% of local American TV news is made up of commercials, weather, sport, chat and 'bear eats popsicle' type fluff; of the part that is news, most concerns crime or disasters. Two-thirds of all media coverage of the Clinton health care reform debate concerned the political battle; only a third looked at the issues. As Hume puts it, on the one hand we are amusing ourselves to death instead of facing common challenges, and on the other, we listen to a coverage of politics that is like a Greek chorus, full of proverbial wisdom and hopelessness. This distorts the nation's understanding of itself.

Leaders like Martin Luther King and Justin Dart have led, rather than followed, public opinion. If they had not done so, history would have stagnated on the issues that have meant so much to them. Nonetheless, there are deep problems with courts deciding policy, or even politicians deciding to pass laws like the ADA, if public support is lacking. It is a problem because it exposes inadequacies in our democracy that can only be addressed by radical change. It is also a problem because, if law is part of a dynamic of change, the rest of the dynamic may be harder to spark into action if the public is ill-informed or unsupportive.

The introduction of the ADA

In the immediate lead-up to the ADA being passed, the disability movement in Washington made a conscious decision to engage in no media coverage. Chief lobbyist Pat Wright said that if the movement had sought press attention, 'we would have been forced to spend half our time trying to teach reporters what's wrong with their stereotypes of people with disabilities'. As it was, they could concentrate on getting the law passed – without risk of its being undermined by negative media reports. The bar on media work was so successful that *New York Times* congressional reporter Steven Holmes commented, after the ADA passed the Senate: 'This bill seemed to come out of nowhere' (quoted in Hartman and Johnson 1993). It was hard to make a story if the key players – the Washington disability community – did not want to say anything.

This was part of an extremely effective strategy to get the Bill passed. Several people within the disability community have expressed surprise that it did pass at this point in history. It was, some said, contingent on the right people being in the right place at the right time. Rather than putting pressure on politicians by working with journalists to highlight issues, the disability community brought disabled people into Congress to give testimony directly. Next, lobbyists suggested that the Bill should have as its proposers only representatives and senators who either were disabled themselves or had a family member who was. This had the extremely powerful effect of encouraging more and more people to 'come out' about their own or their relatives' disability. Suddenly, decision makers were telling stories of what it was like to carry a brother up the steps of a synagogue or to care for a psychiatrically disabled daughter. This undermined the Bill's opponents. If they criticised the disability lobby, it was now clear that they were criticising, at an almost personal level, people such as Senator Bob Dole or Senator Tom Harkin.

The strategy also involved the grassroots mobilization of disability activists, who lobbied key Congressional representatives, and negotiations in Washington with representatives and their research staff. The whole enterprise was described by its key co-ordinators in military terms: the 'general' decided on strategy, and the troops executed it. Everyone had a clearly allocated area of responsibility, and lobbyists and grassroots activists met daily to plan. The result was that an extraordinary level of alliance was built up: between Republicans and Democrats, between labour, business and the disability community. Coalitions were built with the Leadership Conference on Civil Rights (the first time the broader civil rights movement had engaged so actively in disability politics) and with gay rights organisations concerned about

AIDS (Watson 1993). The rhetoric used to support the law gives a flavour of the level of unity apparently achieved:

> Throughout our nation's history, our disabled citizens have not been provided the opportunity to participate in all phases of society. Designed to provide 43 million Americans with enhanced opportunity this bill, then embodies the conservative ideal of equal opportunity (Newt Gingrich, US House of Representatives, 22 May 1990).

> The ADA means inclusion, integration, and empowerment. For business, it means more customers, increased profits, and additional qualified workers. For labor, it means greater protection from arbitrary action for members. And for government, it means more taxpayers and fewer persons dependent on welfare, social security and other social programs (Senator Tom Harkin 1994).

The disability spokespeople constantly nurtured this sense of win–win for everyone:

> The enemy is not civil rights or free enterprise; it is not business or labor or people with disabilities – there is no enemy here today (Justin Dart, quoted in ADA Summit 1990).

Meetings repeatedly brought all interested parties, from business to disability rights activists, to the same table. Britain, by contrast, only began to embark on major cross-interest discussions some years after the DDA was passed, with the formation in 1997 of a Ministerial Disability Rights Task Force.

Much play was made of the patriotic notion that America was leading the world, taking a step that was morally, as well as economically, sound:

> America's greatest export has been its concept of human rights. Let us continue that tradition with this bill (Senator Bob Dole, US Senate, 16 July 1993).

> Five years ago today I had the privilege of signing into law the ADA... Together we brought a shameful wall of exclusion tumbling down. Together we did the right thing (George Bush, statement sent to Justin Dart, 26 July 1995).

This bipartisan acceptance of the 'win–win' construction of the Act's probable effect was an achievement that cannot be overestimated. The ADA was overwhelmingly passed in the House by 377 votes to 28, and in the Senate by 91 to 6. Nevertheless, some issues have arisen in public and political debate since the law was introduced, which raise questions about how agreement is or can be reached and how the public is or can be involved.

A new public debate: the attack on the ADA

From 1994, when the Republicans swept into power in Congress, it was argued that the ADA was imposing huge costs on business and being used by people who were not disabled at all. 'Perhaps most tragically the ADA may cause employer hostility towards the disabled', stated Edward Hudgins of the right-wing Cato Institute. He picked a few atypical cases to show how absurd ADA claims are, arguing that businesses that have suffered as a result should be compensated and that the ADA itself should be changed or repealed (Hudgins 1995).

Edward Hudgins has said that benevolence in the US towards black people had been eroded because people now think that they get jobs through special favours; the same would happen to disabled people. Already, he said, 'a lot of businessmen would not say this publicly, but they try never to hire a handicapped person because they see a lawsuit waiting to happen' (personal communication 1996). The answer was to replace the entitlement society with private benevolence on the part of individuals and companies. Some companies were hiring disabled people, and they were more likely to do so without laws to deter them.

Also in 1995, the Heritage Foundation published a collection of 'regulatory horror stories', under the title *Strangled by Red Tape* (Heritage Foundation 1995). Most of the chapter on 'feelgood legislation' was devoted to the ADA. It cites examples such as a bank making drive-by cash machines accessible to blind people, and an obese person being covered by the ADA. Since this is explicitly a list of horror stories, there is no need to justify the selection of cases, but they do misrepresent the law, arguing for example that it is the employee who decides whether he or she is disabled (when in fact a functional test is involved). They state that the ADA has meant high costs and therefore job losses – although they offer no evidence – and that those getting 'rewards' from the ADA 'are often not disabled at all. They are simply opportunistic parasites who live off the profits and hard work of others'. The EEOC uses this 'newest weapon of choice... to destroy companies and discourage entrepreneurship'.

The disability community had argued for voluntary agreements for years, with no response. It was only with the passage of the Rehabilitation Act 1973 and the ADA that they began to see change (Shapiro 1993). But the Cato Institute and the Heritage Foundation had very strong links into both Congress and the media. By 1995, Newt Gingrich had reversed his view that the ADA embodied the conservative ideal of equal opportunity (see above) and was calling it a regulatory nightmare.

There are various views on why the carefully constructed bipartisan alliance on the ADA began to fracture. Hudgins believes that the business community never really supported it; they saw that they were bound to lose, because of Bush's support, so they 'had to rush in to negotiate the terms of surrender'. Hudgins does not believe that the terms of the ADA protect business: 'the concept of undue hardship reminds me of Chamberlain saying "peace in our time". It is not worth the paper it is written on' (personal communication 1996).

This, however, is contradicted by other evidence. There was no upsurge of objection from employers: survey data showed that most employers continued to support the ADA (as discussed in Ch. 8). Some employers undoubtedly supported the Cato Institute line ('the ADA? Oh yes, the Full Employment for Lawyers Act') or thought it was something that made them into victims ('it'll take a while for people to feel this isn't something that makes them lose out'), but there were no data to suggest major problems. Court decisions have, if anything, applied narrow definitions on who counts as 'disabled', and companies are not charged any compensatory damages unless they are found guilty of wilful discrimination (see Chs 8 and 9).

The problem for the disability community was that this was not a battle about disability policy but an attack on the role of big government. The analysts at the Cato Institute and the Heritage Foundation writing on the ADA were not disability specialists: they wrote equally on the absurdities of current systems for regulating water standards or drug licensing. The politicians in Congress whom they convinced were equally ideological. If the disability community engaged in a debate on which policies would be most effective, they were faced with people who did not believe that government had a role at all.

This is an example of what communications specialists call a 'moral conflict' (Freeman *et al.* 1992): the parties disagree not only on the substance of an issue, but also on the criteria by which they might judge which arguments are right. For right-wing Republicans, the criterion is whether a given proposal will reduce the role of government; for disability activists it is whether it will have positive effects for disabled people. Moral conflicts are the kind that can lead to violence outside the abortion clinic. Each time one side says something to support its argument – for example, that disabled people's lives have only improved with national civil rights – that just proves to the other side how wrong the first group is, because to them the whole idea of federal civil rights is a marker of a society gone wrong.

In a pure moral conflict, ways forward involve, first, making it apparent. For example, one might say to the media that we could have a society with little regulation and no national civil rights, and spell out the consequences of that, or we could have one with national civil rights and some regulation. This approach was used to an extent by the EEOC when another conflict – between Congress and the President over the budget – closed the government down in early 1996. The EEOC told the media: 'discrimination did not also go on furlough'. Without the EEOC, people dying of AIDS were not getting their claims dealt with; others were losing their jobs because of missing legal deadlines. The implication to readers was 'you may think you want federal government reduced, but take a look at the consequences'.

The second approach in a moral conflict is to try to reach another level of debate, one above the terrain of deadlock. The disability community tried this too. In discussions about research priorities, activists proposed producing a guide for journalists and Congress on how to read evidence on the ADA. Instead of putting out another document saying how effective the ADA is, which would be countered in different terms by the anti-ADA lobby, the idea was to give decision makers and journalists access to a meta-language, a way of making sense of the different research data and arguments that would be put before them.

Another proposal was to seek some consensus on indicators of success of the ADA, to avoid an endless repetition of the claim that the ADA is highly effective, or totally disastrous, depending on viewpoint. Moral conflicts do tend to get as polarised as that: it begins to seem dangerous to tell a more complex truth, to say, for example, that the ADA may be helping people with milder impairments more than others – because that is handing ammunition to the other side. It becomes dangerous even to do research lest the findings contain even one point that can be used by opponents. Unsurprisingly in this climate, the imagery of battle remains strong: disability activists are exhorted to go out and fight. 'No soldier ever died for a more worthy cause', as Justin Dart put it in 1996.

Luckily, the moral conflict does not permeate the whole of political debate. Many politicians, including President Clinton, remained as committed through the 1990s as when the ADA was passed. This enabled the disability community to take action outside the moral conflict, to build support. For example, in 1995 a journalist, Rick Kahler, wrote an article for the *Rapid City Journal* attacking the 'regulatory black hole' of the ADA (2 April 1995). He was then subjected to an extremely respectful form of lobbying by Justin Dart and others – letters beginning 'Rick Kahler is a good writer, a good businessman, and a good citizen, but he has gotten a bum steer about the ADA... from sources that he should be able to trust' and so forth. Kahler became convinced that he had made errors, and said so in a subsequent article headed 'I blew it on the ADA' (17 September 1995). At the end of the year, Kahler cited his education by the disability community as a high spot of 1995.

Disability activists have effectively lobbied political decision makers. In 1996, the Mayor of Philadelphia stated in the media that costs prohibited putting in kerb cuts, his figures having already been established in Court to be exaggerated. A meeting of disability activists, coincidentally taking place that day, was wondering, 'why are we sitting here talking?' 'Let's go challenge the Mayor of Philadelphia', said someone. 'OK,' said the chair, 'who's coming?' Within a couple of hours, a group of disabled people had formed a line inside the Hilton Hotel, where a Conference of Mayors was meeting, and set up a chant, filmed all the while by TV crews there for the conference. As hotel staff dealt with the situation immaculately – no one wants the bad publicity of disrespect to disabled people – the President of the Conference of Mayors emerged. Put on the spot by disability leader Becky Ogle, he pledged on camera the Mayors' full support for the ADA. This was a step beyond the moral conflict, achieved by approaching people who were not entirely anti-regulation and putting pressure on them to say so.

Despite the strategic ability and flair of Washington's disability community, they were faced with the legacy of the decision not to work with the media when the ADA was being passed. This left the path clear for those who opposed the ADA to set the stories running, leaving disability activists on the defensive. While they did try to pre-empt the kinds of criticism that have been levelled at the ADA – by stating that they wanted harmonious compliance, with minimal cost and litigation – they did less to initiate completely new 'narratives'. The coverage of the ADA that occurred between 1988 and 1993 did show signs of a paradigm shift from pity to rights, both sometimes being present in the same article (Haller, undated). The public, however, still knew relatively little of the ADA until they were told that it was a 'regulatory nightmare'.

If – and it is a big if – at that historical moment the disability movement had been able to seize the initiative in public discourse, they would not have had to worry about 'moral conflict' to the same degree. Groups in powerful positions in public debate do not mind whether their opponents attack them vigorously. They either play to win or build consensus to shore up their position; they are not obliged to build bridges to be heard.

As it was, the anti-regulation view began to take hold as a key narrative. Once a narrative is in place, it seems like common sense. It may make employers more afraid of the ADA – in the absence of sound information on the law. The employers' reluctance to take on disabled people then becomes a self-fulfilling prophecy.

Many people use the term 'backlash' for the attack on the ADA, following Faludi's analysis of the earlier 'backlash' against feminism (Faludi 1991). 'Backlash' has become an overused term: it implies it is only a response to actions taken by feminists or disabled people. This does give the disability community some credit for having achieved change, but it risks blaming the victim. In 1987, Sutherland wrote, under the headline 'Backlash', 'all is not well in our movement. In our struggle for dignified, meaningful lives, we've alienated able-bodied people'. The implication is that the response of able-bodied people is entirely the responsibility of those who are disabled, and that disabled people should, to return to Martin Luther King's dilemma, have waited rather than pushed too far too fast. The so-called 'backlash' is a forelash – a clearly articulated policy based on an equally clear philosophy. History suggests that, if a social movement avoids confrontation and 'fits in', it will not necessarily be accepted.

It is vital to analyse which strategies will achieve objectives – and sometimes not to confront at a particular moment. However, it is risky to assume that if only one conforms, attack – or 'backlash' – can be avoided. Proactive work with the public is also important to assure the credibility of lobbying organisations. While one advocate told me that 'to have influence in Washington you just show up', there are constant attacks on interest groups for lack of accountability. The disability community has built a national grassroots movement partly in response to these concerns. Additionally, social movements have looked enviously at the mailing list size and strength of organisations such as the Christian Coalition.

The ADA is a rather extraordinary law for having relied so heavily on insider politics – and having won. It cannot, however, be assumed that insider politics will in future suffice.

All the dilemmas about how to safeguard the ADA are magnified when it comes to the interests of mental health user/survivors in particular.

The attack on 'psychiatric disability'

Over 160 organisations concerned with disability or health supported the ADA and achieved considerable solidarity:

> No subgroup of people with any type of physical or mental disability, or perceived disability, no matter how politically impotent or how stigmatised, will be sacrificed (Task Force 1990).

Although mental health user/survivors were not heavily involved in the lobbying effort, the Bazelon Center for Mental Health Law played a key role in helping to keep psychiatric disability in the Act. There were those who wanted it excluded. Senator Jesse Helms went through the DSM (and his own imagination) and asked a long series of questions in the Senate about who would be covered by the Bill, beginning as follows:

Mr Helms:	Does the list of disabilities include pedophiles?
Mr Harkin:	What?
Mr Helms:	P-e-d-o-p-h-i-l-e-s?
Mr Harkin:	I can assure the Senator, no.
Mr Helms:	How about schizophrenics?
Mr Harkin:	Schizophrenics, yes.
Mr Helms:	Kleptomania?
Mr Harkin:	Well, I am not certain on that.
Mr Helms:	Manic depressives?
Mr Harkin:	Manic depressives, yes, I can state that…
Mr Helms:	Homosexuals?
Mr Harkin:	No; absolutely not…

Mr Helms: A schizophrenic is covered, the Senator said. I want
to know if an adoption agency is forbidden to take
that into consideration if the prospective adopter is
a schizophrenic or manic depressive.

Mr Harkin: I am sure there are plenty of manic depressives in
this country – I know some. I have met some who
are completely controlled... Each case would have
to be handled on its own merits...

Mr Helms: If this were a bill involving people in a wheelchair
or those who have been injured in the war, that is
one thing... But how did you get into the business
of classifying people who are HIV positive, most of
whom are drug addicts or homosexuals or bisexu-
als, as disabled? (ADA Senate Floor Debate, 7
September 1989).

And so it went on. Clearly, the conflation of mental disorder with
moral turpitude (see Ch. 3), and the sharp division between
deserving disabilities (war wounds and wheelchair use) and undeserving (mental disorders and AIDS) had not died by 1989 – at least
not in the US Congress.

Unsurprisingly, mental health barely featured in positive discussion of the ADA in Congress or the media. Although some testimony presented in Congress concerned people with mental health
problems, far more concerned people with mobility or sensory
impairments. In the media coverage that did occur on the ADA,
6.9% concerned people with mental health problems and 48%
people using wheelchairs (Haller, undated). Vaccaro notes that
literature on workplace accommodations also focused more on
people with physical than mental impairments (Vaccaro 1991).

While it was a huge achievement to keep mental health in the
ADA at all, once there it was almost off the map in public debate.
This made it easy for ADA critics to say later that the law was being
used by a group – those with psychiatric problems – for whom
Congress had never intended it. The public did not know any
better. If Shapiro's point that the ADA was leading rather than
following public opinion was true in general, it was hugely more
true for people diagnosed mentally ill.

When the Cato Institute and the Heritage Foundation began
their attacks on the ADA, they singled out psychiatric disability as
the area 'open to the greatest abuse' (Hudgins 1995). The cases that
Hudgins cites to damn the ADA are virtually all mental health

cases, and highly atypical, for example, that of the dentist who claimed he had harassed patients because of a disability and the employee who claimed disability after he was fired for bringing a gun to work. It is notable that the same few absurd cases get used again and again as though they were emblematic of the ADA itself. People bringing such cases have not won in the courts, a fact that does not deter Hudgins from arguing that 'many kinds of aberrant behavior that previously might have cost an employee his job now merit ADA coverage'.

The press drew on the same few outlandish examples. Article after article looked at the supposed requirement to employ people who might be violent (*Wall Street Journal*, 19 July 1994 and see Figure 10.1 depicting a service user as an axeman), at supposed coverage for 'chronic lateness syndrome' (*Washington Post*, 4 July 1995) and at the need to get away from being a 'victim nation'. In 1996, George Will wrote in the *Washington Post* that 'if you are just slightly offensive your rights will not kick in. But if you are seriously insufferable to colleagues at work, you have a right not to be fired.' Now the 'colossal jerk' was protected, in a process of medicalising what society used to see as faults of mind and character (*Washington Post*, 4 April 1996).

Politicians also saw this as an easy way of attacking the ADA. Newt Gingrich and Dick Armey, in *Restoring the Dream: The Bold New Plan by House Republicans* wrote:

> Who could be against providing civil-rights protections and special accommodations for those in our society who are blind or in wheelchairs? But under the Act, 43 million people are potentially considered disabled... the list includes drug abusers, the obese and the emotionally disturbed (Gingrich and Armey 1994).

This onslaught on psychiatric disability is partly explained as a wedge issue. ADA critics knew that people with psychiatric disabilities were vulnerable because they had less public support than, for example, wheelchair users. We have not established in the public's mind a piece of common sense to the effect that there are people who have real psychiatric impairments and who can work. Two competing narratives in the public debate say that they are either 'berserkers' and dangerous (in which case they should not be in the workplace at all) or malingerers, people who are 'jerks' who should just take personal responsibility. There is barely a glimpse of a middle ground, of people qualified to work and disabled

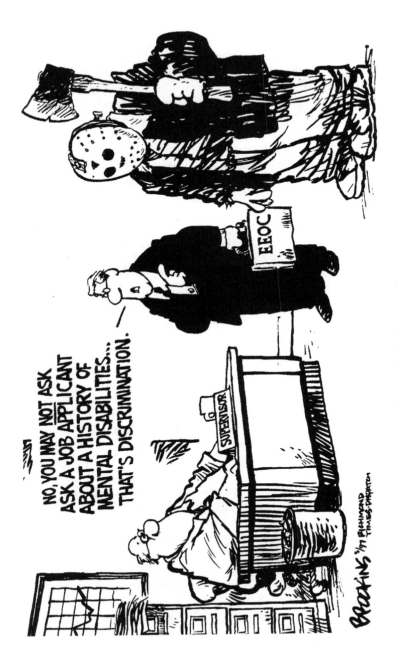

Figure 10.1 Cartoon depicting a service user as an axeman

enough to need protective laws. This may possibly also explain judges' tendency to see people either as too disabled to be qualified or too qualified to be disabled (as discussed in Ch. 9).

Edward Hudgins of the Cato Institute told me that, while he would like to see the ADA abolished altogether, he would, if we had to have it, draw the line at people with mental health problems. Speaking of the 'therapy society', he said:

> I want to shake people who say, I just can't go to work, man. If I were someone with a real disability – like Stephen Hawking – I'd resent being put on the same level as some whining ne'er do well like that. People with a handicap really can't help it – they didn't poke their own eyes out. It dilutes the concern for real disability if you muddy the waters with these people who have a 'syndrome'.

When pressed about whether he thought anyone might have a 'real' psychiatric disability, he said, 'maybe if it is a biologically based disability and it affects them on the job – but then maybe they shouldn't be on the job anyway'.

It seems that people with mental health problems are still not seen as 'innocent' in the same way as other disabled people are (see discussion in Ch. 7), that anyone who does not accept a biological understanding should not be protected (see Ch. 4), and that 'real' disability is incompatible with work. These ideas make rights elusive indeed.

The response to the attack on the coverage of psychiatric disability from the disability community was a confirmation of unity. Justin Dart responded to Newt Gingrich and Dick Armey's points in the following terms:

> Mr Speaker, these are cheap shots, direct appeals to the very prejudice that the ADA was designed to eliminate… Fact: abusers of illegal drugs are not protected by the ADA… Fact: 'the emotionally disturbed' form by far the largest segment of the disability community… They suffer the most profound prejudice and vicious discrimination. Your public suggestion that their civil rights should not be protected is frightening. It reinforces prejudice and seems to condone the devastating rejections of their humanity that people with psychiatric disabilities suffer every day (letter from Justin Dart to Newt Gingrich, 4 June 1995).

The Washington disability community did not try to dissociate itself from the 'crazies' as some mental health user/survivors had long charged. Paul Steven Miller, Commissioner of the EEOC with responsibility for disability, warned publicly of the danger of people with psychiatric disabilities being picked off (Miller 1995). The principle of keeping all types of disability in the Act, no matter how stigmatised, still held in the late 1990s. Judi Chamberlin described the attack on mental health survivors as a wolf circling a group of sheep, picking out those that were weakest. Thus, the mental health user/survivor movement became more deeply involved with the ADA.

The attack on psychiatric disability posed certain dilemmas for the disability and mental health movements. Some thought it preferable, in order to safeguard the ADA, not to raise further the profile of mental health and the ADA. If statements came only from the broader disability community, this would both demonstrate afresh the unity between groups and avoid giving opponents a further platform to debate mental health specifically. Politicians would be reluctant to be seen to attack disabled people in general – especially if they gained news coverage in their wheelchairs. Old notions of pity adhering to physically – but not psychiatrically – disabled people made them hard to attack.

However, 'keeping quiet' about mental health could entrench the problem of lack of public knowledge of, and support for, fair access for user/survivors. A combination of proactive media and educational work from an all-disability perspective – to safeguard law – and from a mental health perspective – to achieve longer-term goals – seems the most promising strategy.

A second dilemma was whether to head into the 'moral conflict' arena using the language of rights, risking attack from those who believed that the entitlement society has caused dependency, crime and assorted other social ills, or to frame arguments in a 'preemptive' way by saying that the ADA would involve minimum cost and litigation, would get people out of the dependency culture and would create savings for business. Adopting only the second approach might create a credibility gap: advocacy organisations are not known for their primary concern for business profits, nor business-backed think tanks, which sometimes argue that scrapping regulation will help disabled people to get jobs, for their primary commitment to disabled people's rights. On the one hand, it is important to find credible ways of demonstrating advantages to business, in particular by identifying business leaders prepared to make the case to their peers (as when the Washington Business Group on Health said that the ADA could reduce the annual $17 billion in lost production through depression). On the other, one must simultaneously frame legitimate demands for rights in terms that will be heard (contribution, fairness and opportunity) rather than pretending to have no rights agenda. Avoiding conflict at all costs can effectively gag disability organisations. Conflict, if it occurs, can also present opportunities as well as risks – to galvanise a movement, to spur action.

The third dilemma was, in promoting examples to the media and politicians of user/survivors able to work but facing discrimination, what types of user/survivor should be profiled. Some thought it vital to include people whom 'middle America' could identify with – those who did not look too strange, who had relatively non-frightening problems (depression, preferably in the past, and not schizophrenia). Yet some grassroots activists were angered by such 'compromises' struck in Washington, which could create another schism between the few 'OK' user/survivors and the others, abandoned even by their own advocacy organisations. For long-term goals, public education clearly needed to highlight a range of different experience (as was discussed in Ch. 5, in the context of the risks of a 'continuum' model neglecting those who are most disabled).

The links to other social and policy areas

Public discourse on the ADA tends to divorce it from other social issues. Haller found that the dominant image of a disabled person in ADA coverage was 'a white middle class man in a wheel-chair' (Haller, undated). The public has not been encouraged to give much thought to the experiences of, for example, blind people of colour, let alone user/survivors of colour.

The lack of attention to intersecting social policy areas means that the ADA may be expected to solve problems, such as high unemployment among disabled people, that a law alone cannot solve. The National Organization on Disability predicted that 2 million unemployed people would find work as a result of the ADA. Senator Bob Dole subsequently suggested setting a target of 8 million by the end of the century (Dole 1994). Overambitious goals for one law can, however, lead to later conclusions that the law has failed. There is a considerable need to complexify debate – to ensure that people consider social security, employment, housing and other policy trends as they intersect with civil rights (as discussed earlier, in Ch. 9).

Not a backlash but a forelash: the British experience

In Britain, there was no disability movement ban on media work, as in the US, but there was little positive media coverage of the law at all, given its deep unpopularity among disabled people (see Ch. 9). Any proactive media work that did occur focused more on wheelchair users than other disabled people, more on white than black people.

The general public has not been made aware that measures to combat discrimination against disabled people include those with mental health problems. By 1996, even opinion leaders – in the media, academia, politics, the civil service and business – thought the following people were not disabled: those with severe facial scarring, those with a speech impediment, and 'a person with depression who found it difficult to make minor changes to their routine'. All are potentially covered by the DDA (National Disability Council 1996).

The British law covers fewer people with less 'traditional' impairments than does the American law. Those with alcohol and drug problems are not included; nor are those with mental disorders that are not 'clinically recognised' (see Ch. 9). This has not, however, stopped the beginning of a British attack on legal protections for people with mental health problems. In 1997, *The Times* reported the American EEOC Guidance on the ADA and psychiatric disability, arguing that the bar on asking prospective employees about a history of schizophrenia or manic depression appeared 'dramatically to increase the scope of the ADA' (1 May 1997). It took a letter from Mind to point out that it was not only strange Americans who outlawed discrimination against psychiatrically disabled people: the British DDA did too (albeit less comprehensively), a fact of which *The Times* was apparently unaware. Also in 1997, a *Daily Telegraph* editorial stated:

> The word 'disabled' calls to mind images of people confined to wheelchairs; yet fewer than 75,000 of the 6.5 million people classed as disabled are in this category. The deep-felt and commendable public sympathy for disabled people can inhibit rational policy making... Was it reasonable to order private businesses to provide equal access at an estimated cost of £20 billion? Are too many able-bodied people claiming benefits intended for the genuinely handicapped? (16 December 1997).

There was no basis for the £20 billion figure. The caution built into the British law has not stopped an attack on people who are not seen as 'genuinely' (that is, physically) disabled. Indeed, it might be argued that excluding many people with mental health problems, and with drug or alcohol problems, has pandered to the prejudiced view that these are not 'real' impairments. Making compromises does not prevent 'backlash' because the so-called backlash is in truth a forelash, which will be expressed anyway, on the basis of political ideology, shared internationally between well-connected think tanks.

There are large differences between the political and cultural landscapes of Britain and the US, for example in public attitudes to litigation, in how the media are funded and controlled, and in lobbying practices. Both, however, share a common problem: they have introduced laws, of different strengths, which aim to counter the discrimination faced by people with mental health problems, among other disabled people; and they have not informed the public – nor even opinion leaders like the London *Times* – of what is happening, why and how it can be effectively implemented. This leaves a vacuum that is readily filled by scaremongers pointing to the costs, and risks to safety, of allowing people with psychiatric problems rights alongside the 'deserving' disabled, who are pityingly portrayed as being 'confined' to their wheelchairs. Moreover, the task of telling the public that people with mental health problems also need legal protections, as disabled people, is not eased by the fact that much of the user/survivor movement – especially in Britain – remains cut off from the disability movement and in some ways still resists the very model (disability inclusion) that offers the most solid grounds for a hope of change in users/survivors' social status (as argued in Ch. 7).

Conclusion

The original bipartisan support for the ADA, the later fragmentation of the alliance, and strategies used by the disability community to offset attack, provide a context in which to understand why the ADA is not a pure 'disability rights' law. It arose, and is interpreted, within a context of contradictory forces, which have sometimes become polarised to the point of major confrontation. Parts of the law emerged from long-standing prejudices: the exclusion of certain 'morally based' disorders (see Ch. 9), for example, occurred because of objections from Senator Jesse Helms and others.

The disability community chose the unusual step of debarring media coverage during the passage of the ADA because they did not trust journalists to present their aims fairly. Their alternative, highly sophisticated, strategy to build political support – through personal testimony from disabled people in Congress and through encouraging politicians to 'come out' about their own and their families' experience of disability – was highly effective in getting the law passed. But it left a legacy. The public knew little of the ADA and less of the fact that it covered people with mental health problems. This left opponents the scope to make sharp impressions on an unknowing public and rendered the task of building the necessary support for implementation difficult.

The disability movement has had some successes in offsetting the attack on the ADA, for example by using 'meta-language' techniques in the face of a 'moral conflict' with ideological opponents. It has achieved less in proactively framing debates, especially in relation to the rights of mental health user/survivors.

The attack on the ADA is best understood as a proactive ideological assault, eased by a lack of public support for user/survivors' rights. It is not a 'backlash' caused by the disability movement pushing 'too far too fast'. In Britain, where government went much less far less fast, the attack still emerged. The attack is a forward-pushing anti-regulatory position. Simple caution on the part of disabled people will not stem it.

The major challenge facing user/survivors, and the disability community generally, in both countries, is how to transform public discourse, thereby changing the way in which policy and law are framed and interpreted; and how to create changes on the ground that enable anti-discrimination work to become a lived reality. User/survivors and allies face a huge stumbling block: opposition to the very idea of inclusion for people with mental health problems. Senator Helms' comments epitomise the established commonsense view that people who are 'manic depressive' or 'schizophrenic' should – obviously – not participate in the workforce or adopt children. That 'common sense' has to be overturned, through both proactive work to change the constructions that people place on mental illness (which will be discussed in Ch. 11) and through local action that creates direct change in how user/survivors and other members of communities interact (discussed in Ch. 12).

CHAPTER 11

Influencing Public Opinion

Identifying effective methods

An almost automatic response from users and service providers to evidence of discrimination on mental health grounds is to call for education, in schools or through the media (Rose 1996). For example:

> People should go on television and explain what it's like. Explain we're just people with a problem (cited in Rose 1996).

However, we know relatively little about which messages, and which methods of conveying or debating them, will prove effective with which groups, in terms of either changing attitudes or, still less, changing behaviour. Literature search after literature search concludes that more evaluations of practical approaches are needed (Bhugra 1989, Link *et al.* 1992, Repper and Brooker 1996, Wolff *et al.* 1996a). One-off media campaigns have not demonstrated significant achievements in terms of attitude or behaviour change (perhaps partly because more negative media messages constantly compete with them; see Ch. 3), although results appear more promising where media campaigns are backed by ongoing community-based education and action (Barker *et al.* 1993, Wolff *et al.* 1996a). Even so, of the few community education programmes that have been fully evaluated, results have been mixed: Cumming and Cumming (1957) and Gatherer and Reid (1963) both found community education to be ineffective.

The history of discriminatory attitudes exerts a powerful influence across generations (see Ch. 3). Bedini (1991) argues that the mad, evil monsters of present-day horror films are very similar to the freak shows of the 1880s when the 'elephant man' or 'Jojo the dog-faced boy' were displayed to a wondering public. Both create an image of a creature that is neither human nor animal to elicit fear and amazement, as does the repeated media reference to mentally ill people 'roaming' the streets – conjuring up images of lions or rabid dogs. We can hardly assume that teaching people a few facts about the nature and prevalence of mental health problems will be sufficient to interrupt this cultural history. We may be able to derail or reroute it, but exactly how is not self-evident.

Writers on negative attitudes towards people with physical impairments have listed numerous sources of prejudice, including a socio-cultural emphasis on the 'body beautiful'; a value placed on economic productivity; the influences of childhood conditioning, which form and set attitudes early; a religious belief that disability is a punishment for sin, leaving the non-disabled person facing survivor guilt – why should he or she not be punished too?; disability as a reminder of vulnerability and death; and many more (Livneh 1982):

> Due to the complexity of the interacting factors which contribute to the creation of negative attitudes... any experimental study of short duration, hoping to change attitudes, is futile at best. Attempts to modify the prevailing negative attitudes have been generally unsuccessful (Livneh 1982).

Attitudes towards people with mental health problems are generally more negative than those towards other disabled people. Yuker (1988) ranked 24 disabilities in terms of their acceptability, as established through a range of empirical studies of public attitudes. Mental illness came 23rd out of 24; only multiple disabilities were viewed more negatively.

Despite some evidence that attitudes towards mental illness have become slightly more positive in the post-war period (Repper and Brooker 1996, Hayward and Bright 1997), some local studies show attitudes unchanged over time (Huxley 1993) – in one case, no improvement in 23 years (D'Arcy and Brockman 1976). In Britain, hardening attitudes in the 1990s appear to be linked to media coverage (see Ch. 2). Fattah identifies a link between discriminatory attitudes and economic insecurity (Fattah 1984).

We do not know exactly how best to mitigate the impact of economic insecurity, to channel fears into directions other than prejudice. Nor do we know 'what are the incentives for the nation to end discrimination against people labelled mentally ill. Economic? Compassion? Concern for social justice?' (Center for Mental Health Services 1995) or how to interrupt the tendency for media and the public to make groups who are already 'other' – such as black people – take on the feared characteristics of stigmatised disease (Joffe 1996).

It is clear from small-scale studies that the messages that the mental health movement believes will change attitudes often simply do not look the same to those who are supposed to have their attitudes changed.

- The mental health community often promotes the idea that mental health and ill-health are on a continuum (see Ch. 5), with no radical break between them, in order to destigmatise all mental health problems.

The public tends to reject the notion of a 'continuum'; indeed, their disbelief caused the failure of a Canadian education campaign (Cumming and Cumming 1957). More recently, the English Health Education Authority's research into young people's attitudes found 'a remarkably consistent conceptual map', which placed everyday emotions and understandable depressions – caused by long-term unemployment or the death of a close relative – on one side of a rigid divide, on the other side of which lay mental illness. The first side was safe, ordinary, predictable, 'full of people like me, people I know'. The other side was mysterious and strange, unpredictable, shocking and frightening, populated by odd people, strangers and misfits (Health Education Authority 1997a).

Jones and Cochrane (1981) and Rogers and Pilgrim (1997) found that lay beliefs among adults conceptualised 'mental illness' as psychosis. For example: 'I don't class depression and things like that as mental illness. "Mentally ill" to me has always conjured up the visions of the slightly deranged, the particular characters that wander round town centres' (Rogers and Pilgrim 1997). Although some studies find that people believe anyone can develop a mental illness (Department of Health 1993), the 'illness' is not seen as continuous with more ordinary problems such as bereavement.

These findings mean that campaigns promoting the continuum idea will not be easy to integrate into people's existing frameworks of thinking and are likely to be rejected. It may be much more promising to test messages promoting the idea that people who are, indeed, different merit respect and humanity, thereby capitalising on the 'pool of goodwill' towards users that has been identified in a number of studies (Wolff *et al.* 1996a, Repper *et al.* 1997).

- The mental health community often assumes that emphasising the commonness of mental health problems – the fact that one in four people experience them in one form or another each year – will destigmatise them.

England's Health Education Authority (1997a) found that young people did not find such statistics credible: 'Don't believe it. No one I know is mental. How can it be one in four. It's like AIDS, they try and scare you about that but I don't know anyone who's got it' (young man). Public opinion research in New Zealand found that a pilot message 'If you have or have had a mental illness you are in good company' made some people think 'there were a lot of dangerous people with mental illness in the community' (Business Research Centre 1997a).

- The mental health community wants to encourage the public to play their part in enabling user/survivors to be part of communities, by adopting positive attitudes.

A piece of New Zealand research found that people were sceptical about the motives for this type of campaign, believing that the government was trying to shirk its responsibilities and offload mentally ill people on to the community – 'softening up the general public before the floodgates were opened' (Business Research Centre 1997a). It might, they thought, be preferable to spend the money on improving mental health services rather than preparing the public to replace them. In Britain, a 1990 survey found that half of those surveyed thought that moving people from hospital into the community was 'just a way that the government can save money' (ICM 1990).

- The mental health community seeks to explain to the public that their attitude can make a real difference.

Some respondents to the New Zealand research saw this as a slight: 'You're telling me that I've got the wrong attitude to begin with. Have I?' People from minority communities thought that their own cultural attitudes were being overridden. For example, Pacific Island people did not like the statement 'The person isn't the illness; the person is living with the illness', because it positioned the person living with the illness in isolation, whereas they conceptualised 'mental illness' in terms of the person's involvement in the community and family (Eru Pomare Maori Health Research Centre 1997a).

This is also a risk in Britain. Wolff *et al.* (1996b) argue for targeting public education towards African and African-Caribbean people because one study found that they had more controlling attitudes towards people with mental health problems than white people. Possible explanations might arguably include poverty, generating a lower tolerance of disruptive behaviour, or discriminatory media coverage, making black people want to hide 'madness' to avoid confirming white prejudices. Certainly, a campaign premised on the need to change the attitudes of black British people – without changes in the discriminatory way in which black people are treated by the media and mental health system (Sashidharan and Francis 1993, Sayce 1995a, Wilson and Francis 1997) – might be met with some resistance.

- The mental health community tends to believe that health promotion efforts emphasising the importance of positive mental health, rather than concentrating on mental illness, will break down fear and stigma.

Rogers and Pilgrim (1997) found that people could not easily articulate what 'positive mental health' was, although they could describe physical health. Therefore 'it may be that efforts to construct a salatogenic [that is, positive health-based] notion of mental health are doomed to failure'. There is no conceptual framework into which such messages can be readily absorbed and integrated, which suggests that further work on the conceptual models and how to communicate them is required if this strategy is to be effectively pursued (Secker 1998). Linking positive mental health to community, rather than just individual, well-being may be most promising (Social Exclusion Unit 1998; see also Ch. 5).

- The mental health community often imagines that messages designed to encourage people to talk about problems will reduce stigma.

Rogers and Pilgrim (1997) found that people often thought that disclosing problems involved 'losing face' or 'making a big deal of it'. They criticised those who disclosed, especially in exhibitionist ways, such as on TV. 'I think it's a load of codswallop really. They talk about their personal problems the way they do and I mean a personal problem is to keep to yourself I feel. Don't make a blababout of yourself.'

While men are especially likely to reject the 'talk about it' message, many women do also (Rogers and Pilgrim 1997, Health Education Authority 1997a). The Health Education Authority cite an 18-year-old girl: 'you get some girls who go on and on about their problems, it's all they can talk about. I don't think it's because they are having a worse time than anyone else but it's like they've got nothing else to say. We just ignore them.' Boys were even more direct: 'If I saw a man in the street crying I'd think it was funny'; and – of a pilot message encouraging young men to talk about mental distress – 'you'd never say, "oh I feel mentally distressed". People'd think you was barmy. If any of my mates said that to me I'd laugh.'

- The mental health community seeks to encourage people not to discriminate in their behaviour.

The Health Education Authority found that young people thought refusing someone insurance or work might well be justified: 'If I had a garage, if I was the owner, I wouldn't give a job to someone who was mental. They might start stealing stuff or being rude to customers. No way.' The New Zealand research reported that people thought this message 'too strong and authoritarian'.

- The mental health community sometimes wants to convey the message that it's OK to be different.

The New Zealand research described how some people found this incredible because 'difference results in discrimination and always will'. Minority communities said things like 'you ask any Maori… any gay… whether it's OK'. Some agreed strongly in principle – but not necessarily in practice. 'There will always be rednecks.'

- The mental health community assumes that people will take an interest in mental health messages.

The HEA and the New Zealand research found that many people saw mental health issues as irrelevant to them: 'it's old people. You never hear of it happening to anyone our sort of age. No one I know is mental'; 'I don't see it as relevant to me… even if I could see it as relevant for me, what could I do about it?'

(Business Research Centre 1997a). In both studies, some pilot approaches were seen as 'wallpaper', not striking enough to gain attention at all.

Despite all these examples of scepticism, and resistance, we should not despair, for a number of reasons. First, while many people may be cynical about messages stemming from government or official bodies, they may be less so if they hear the message from someone they are already inclined to trust. The most credible presenters of new ideas on disability generally are disabled people who themselves portray non-stereotyped images (Rapier *et al.* 1972, Evans 1976, Ralph 1989). Public attitudes also tend to change when people meet mental health user/survivors. Wolff *et al.* (1996a) found that neighbours of a supported housing project changed their views more through meeting users than through either meeting staff, or receiving educational materials. Brockington *et al.* (1993) and Taylor and Dear (1981) found that people with the least fear of people with mental illness included those with personal or professional experience of mental illness. People may also be inclined to take their peers more seriously than officialdom. For example, a video on mental health made by Finnish students, and distributed with teachers' lesson plans to all local schools catering for 15–16-year-olds, appears to have had a positive impact (World Mental Health Day 1997).

Contact with user/survivors and disabled people changes attitudes positively in some circumstances more than others: when contact is structured, for example planned teaching sessions by disabled people (Ralph 1989); when people's emotions as well as their thinking are affected by the interaction (Clore and Jeffery 1972); and when the non-users see people with schizophrenia as being 'like me' (Levey and Howells 1995), a finding suggesting that enhancing positive attitudes may be as helpful as reversing negative ones, although since the greatest change tends to occur in those who initially have strong negative views, tackling negative attitudes is also worthwhile.

It is possible that the Health Education Authority and New Zealand messages might have had greater impact had those presenting the pilot ideas themselves been user/survivors, who confounded people's initial stereotypes, and used methods that were both structured and prompted an emotional, empathetic response.

Second, we know that there have been some extremely effective campaigns to reframe an issue through activism. The campaign for a deaf President at Gallaudet University (for deaf people), for example, met huge resistance from a University that portrayed deaf student activists as trouble makers. The students succeeded both in their immediate goal – of deposing a non-deaf President in favour of a deaf one – and in achieving a new, civil rights conception of the issues, which 4 years later still permeated University statements and media coverage. A student leader's early comment that 'things will never, never be the same' was borne out as the University consistently and publicly took pride in having done the 'right' thing (that is, the thing it tried not to do) (Barnarrt and Christiansen 1992).

The presence of resistance does not mean that it is impossible to change attitudes but rather that one should avoid a naïve position that 'informing' people of the 'truth' will achieve change. One has to understand people's current views, their motivations – if any – for change and the potential ways of enhancing those motivations, of challenging resistance and of framing the issues to maximise the chance of integrating them into people's existing thinking.

Most campaigns in the mental health field have some limitations on their impact because they do not take all these steps. An evaluation of the British Defeat Depression campaign found that although 69% of GPs surveyed were aware of the campaign, 75% of these said that it had made no difference to their clinical practice. The campaign did not stand out enough from the mass of paper they dealt with and although some GPs followed campaign advice – notably to prescribe antidepressants for longer and in higher doses – others (32%) already felt confident in their diagnosis and management of depression (Macaskill *et al.* 1997). Anecdotal evidence suggests that some GPs objected to psychiatrists telling them how to organise treatment (although they might have been more receptive to messages stemming solely from fellow GPs). Some GPs, like the New Zealand respondents cited above, seemed to think that a campaign aiming to change their views and behaviour implied that their current views had been found wanting, and they therefore ignored the campaign.

Third, we are accumulating knowledge of how different groups of people think about mental health and mental illness, and about which methods are most likely to be effective in creating change.

Starting from people's current attitudes

In 1993, a review of attitude research commented:

A potent mixture of fear, prejudice, enlightened interest and total confusion continue to characterise public responses to mental distress (DVL Associates 1993).

On the one hand, the public in both the US and UK has been found generally to believe that people with mental illness are not a burden on society, that mental illness is not caused by a lack of self-discipline or willpower (Department of Health 1993, Repper and Brooker 1996) and that we need to develop far more tolerant attitudes – 90% held the last view in Britain in 1997 (Department of Health 1997). These opinions, however, coincide with much less accepting attitudes, often in the same respondents. The 1993 Department of Health survey found that 30% thought anyone with a history of mental problems should be excluded from public office, and 43% thought that most women who were once patients in a mental hospital could not be trusted as baby sitters. A 1997 survey on attitudes to schizophrenia found strong support for community care services, but only 13% would be happy if their son or daughter were going out with someone with schizophrenia. More positively, only 18% said that they were unwilling to work alongside someone with schizophrenia (Mori 1997).

The contradictions partly reflect varying methodologies and interpretative frameworks, and partly actual, and unsurprising, complexities of opinion. Public education strategies need to begin from a recognition of contradictions, and to identify opportunities for both building on positive views and neutralising or re-routing negative ones.

Bogdan and Taylor (1989) examine the characteristics of those non-disabled people who do *not* stigmatise disabled people: they tend to view disabled people as reciprocating, not taking; to attribute thinking and individuality to the disabled person; and to see them as having a 'social place'. This suggests that a key way of extending positive attitudes may be to profile a range of different individuals who are contributing. The very low resistance to working alongside someone with schizophrenia (see above) suggests that showing that user/survivors undertake paid and voluntary work is a particularly promising starting point.

Wolff *et al.* (1996a) argue that the pool of goodwill they identified can be channelled. Their local education initiative achieved significant increases in contact between neighbours and service users, when compared with a control area, and in some cases led to friendships. We also need to channel negative views in new directions. If people are afraid of violent crime, we might try engaging with victims' and community groups, and the media, to focus concern where it belongs – mainly on people who are not diagnosed with a mental illness (see Ch. 1). Rather than contextualising homicide by stating that most user/survivors are not violent (true though that is), we should engage with the public's fear (for if we deny it, frightened people are likely to discount our whole message), but route the fear in a direction that fits the facts, away from scapegoats and stereotypes.

Public attitude campaigns also need to account for the ways in which different cultures conceptualise mental health and illness. Since Samoan people see 'mental ill-health' in spiritual and social/collective terms (see above), there might be no need for a campaign emphasising social inclusion: it could not be conceived otherwise. People, however, might be seen as 'ill' because of an ancestor's wrongdoing and thus be viewed negatively (Eru Pomare Maori Health Research Centre 1997a). This suggests a need to work from within the community to reduce blame within this frame of reference, without imposing individualised ideas of 'illness' as the only way in which to dispense with shame.

In Britain, Asian people are sometimes frustrated by white assumptions that Asians 'somatise' mental health problems: they may instead see them as spiritual issues, to be taken to a religious leader rather than a GP (Webb-Johnson 1991). There is discrimination within Asian communities, as everywhere. As Awaz, a Manchester-based Asian mental health group put it, 'The way we are tackling this is to create a community within a community. We hope that this community [of Asian users] will become a force in itself and slowly dismantle the big wall that is created between the community and users who declare that they have mental health problems' (Awaz Group 1997).

In the broader British public, there is a common, and apparently growing (Huxley 1993), belief that mental health problems are caused by social and economic, rather than biological, forces (Rogers and Pilgrim 1997). For example:

> All the problems on them pages [the interviewer's schedule about mental health problems] are to do with money (Rogers and Pilgrim 1997).

Some campaigns have sought to 'correct' these lay views. The Defeat Depression Campaign, having ascertained that the public viewed depression in social terms, to be treated with counselling, put out messages including the value of antidepressants. They were conveying two separate ideas: depression is more biological than you think, and it's OK to seek help. It may be easier to convey only one message, which fits people's existing frame of reference, for example, for anti-discrimination work, 'money worries, grief, unemployment – all can contribute to mental ill health. Don't the casualties deserve a chance to rebuild their lives?'

Studies tend to find that women hold more tolerant attitudes towards user/survivors than do men (Repper and Brooker 1996) and that the most intolerant age groups are older people (Repper and Brooker 1996) and adolescents, especially young men (Brockington *et al.* 1993, Health Education Authority 1997a). The exception to middle-aged tolerance is parents, who are particularly likely to express fearful and controlling views, linked specifically to fears for their own children (Repper and Brooker 1996, Wolff *et al.* 1996b). There is some evidence that tolerant attitudes are more common in people with higher levels of education and higher socio-economic positions (Repper and Brooker 1996) – although some research has found the reverse. Dear (1992) characterises the typical opponent of community mental health facilities as male, well-educated, professional, married, a home owner and living in the suburbs, but Repper *et al.* (1997) found that 'nimby' campaigns occurred equally in affluent suburbs and poor estates.

We should not make assumptions about class differences in intolerance but rather engage different socio-economic groups in debate and test messages with them.

Promoting new constructions

If one-off public education messages – single TV advertisements or posters – may be met with cynicism or boredom (see above), setting new 'narratives' running, through arts or media, may be more promising. We know that the media does influence thinking on mental health (Philo *et al.* 1993) and that films featuring disabled people can have positive (Byrd 1988) as well as negative (Hafer and Narcus 1979) effects. Film is most powerful when accompanied by participant involvement (Ralph 1989).

This knowledge has been translated into action. In Vancouver, Bruce Saunders, who has a diagnosis of manic depression, created 'Movie Monday', showing films on mental health themes inside a local psychiatric hospital. The events, attended by members of the public, user/survivors and mental health workers from outside as well as inside the hospital, are followed by discussion. 'Bruce Saunders first went to the Eric Martin Pavilion [the local psychiatric ward] as a suicidal patient. The place will never be the same', as the local newspaper put it (*Monday Magazine*, 8–14 May 1997).

Similarly, Professor Kay Jamison has put on concerts with orchestras that include players with mental health problems, as well as local chamber music evenings featuring a video on user/survivor musicians followed by debate.

Initiatives evoking powerful emotion or humour can avoid the boredom trap (see above) and provide a counterweight to the scare and power of the 'psycho-killer' images or the humour directed against 'crazy' people (Wahl 1995); facts alone are weak tools. Aidan Shingler makes highly unusual conceptual art from experiences of madness. In one work, he places wine glasses filled with water in a huge circle, on a large picture of the entire globe, and writes:

> I believed that the moon was directly controlling my mind. The thinking behind this belief was as follows: the moon affects the oceans, the sea is of course water, and human beings are composed of 80% water. Therefore my deduction was that the moon affects mind and body. During this phase I drank enormous quantities of H_2O (Shingler 1996).

The viewer is drawn into the unusual logic, which Shingler sets against very ordinary objects in ways that make 'mad' thinking seem in a sense plausible, everyday, yet simultaneously jarring to so-called 'common sense'. The results are 'poignant, inexplicably beautiful' and sometimes 'very funny' (Guardian, 22 August 1997). His work was sold to the Glasgow Museum of Modern Art and viewed in Durham Cathedral by an estimated 10,000 people.

While the mental health movement has been wary of humour, one user-written, award-winning BBC drama was rapturously received by other user/survivors – and by the public. *Taking Over the Asylum*, a 1995 comedy focusing on a radio station run by users inside a psychiatric hospital, succeeded in pointing up the absurdity of the treatment of user/survivors in ways that engaged viewers empathetically with the 'mad'.

Books recounting personal experiences of mental health problems have the power to create understanding through empathy and are becoming big business. These include journalist Tracy Thompson's account of depression (Thompson 1995), shorter pieces by Salman Rushdie and Fay Weldon (Dunn *et al.* 1996), and Kay

Jamison's *An Unquiet Mind*, which reached the *New York Times* best-seller list in 1995 (Jamison 1995). Those stressing the value of professional help appear to be more marketable than those – such as *Call Me Crazy* (Shimrat 1997) or *Beyond Bedlam* (Grobe 1995) – which are more critical of the power of mental health professionals. Jamison's book, however, does touch powerfully on how discrimination operates when mental health professionals find one of 'their own' affected (Jamison 1995).

Soap operas and TV dramas have taken up anti-discrimination themes. In 1996, *Peak Practice* – a British prime-time TV series – carried a story line about a doctor's wife who developed manic depression. It was intended that she would commit suicide. Following lobbying from mental health charities, the programme makers decided that this 'not very positive' message might provoke a bad reaction among viewers (*Daily Record*, 2 January 1998). Instead the wife – an attractive and popular character – faced her husband's shame head on, confronting him in a powerful scene about his reluctance for others to know of her diagnosis. In 1998, pregnant, she grappled with dilemmas of possible termination and the effects of medication on the fetus; for the first time on British TV, access to parenting became a mainstream issue for millions of viewers. The actress playing the part, Yolanda Vazquez, stated that she was proud to have created a character who helped to take the stigma away from mental illness (*Daily Record*, 2 January 1998).

Groups have established the waste of discrimination as an engrossing 'narrative' in news and current affairs. Mind's surveys on discrimination (1996) and 'nimby' campaigns (1997) between them gained over 300 mentions in national and local media. This began to locate user/survivors as the victims rather than the perpetrators of crime. Similarly, one user interviewed in North Carolina about local murders stated, 'I hope nothing like that ever happens to me', neatly overturning the assumption that it is user/survivors who are killers. When asked 'do you think you could ever do anything like that?', the user replied 'No, ma'am!' (Mayer and Barry 1992).

Prime-time documentaries have sometimes conveyed user/survivors' own perspectives on issues usually defined for them by 'experts'. In a 1997 Mental Health Media production, *From the Ashes*, the one woman interviewed, who had been incarcerated in Broadmoor, seemed to undo every stereotype of Broadmoor patients as monsters. Multiple discrimination has, however, been featured far less – and often only on late-night shows.

In 1998, with welfare-to-work high on the British government's agenda, *The Times* portrayed Pathfinder NHS Trust's policy of recruiting users and ex-users as staff in their mental health services. One said, 'when I saw the job advertisement stating that you had to have experience of mental health problems, I thought it was a joke... I love the work. It provides me with security. The patients I work with know about me and they like it. They see what I have achieved and it gives them hope.' Those quoted had diagnoses of manic depression and paranoid schizophrenia. This was a new narrative, suggesting that even the most feared types of mental health problem need not stop people from active citizenship (*The Times*, 7 July 1997). Research suggests the public is much more open to working alongside user/survivors than to more intimate contact, such as personal relationships or letting user/survivors look after one's children (Business Research Centre 1997b); this type of coverage has the potential to extend and give shape to this tolerance.

In order for user/survivors to speak to the media, they need training and support. Some have had only their 'pitiable story' included, while their solid opinions are edited out. In Britain, Mindlink (a user/survivor network) and Mental Health Media have developed guidance and training.

Some one-off public education campaigns have drawn on the knowledge of what the public already believes, challenged the more discriminatory views and extended positive strands. The Australian government produced materials, from 1995, including a poster of a footballer scoring, with the caption 'The defence didn't stop him. Neither did mental illness' (Figure 11.1). Another portrayed a woman serving in a shop, with the caption 'Her customers don't know she has a mental illness. Her workmates couldn't care less.' The material could possibly be faulted for implying that people with mental health problems are 'the same' as everyone else, but initial evaluations did show positive changes in public attitude (cited in New Zealand Ministry of Health 1997).

In Britain, in 1997, the Health Education Authority and Mind distributed bold postcards targeting young people, depicting attractive faces with terms such as 'nutter', 'mental' and 'psycho' written across them, in order to create a sense of disjunction and convey the message 'Why use labels when they don't fit?' Each card gave the background to 'who's really behind the label',

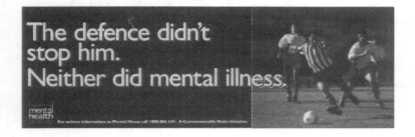

Figure 11.1 Australian Government poster

explaining distress in terms of bereavement, relationship break-down or emerging mental health problems (Figures 11.2a and b). Early feedback suggested that the cards were very well received and were effective in triggering debate.

In the US, the Substance Abuse and Mental Health Services Administration (SAMHSA) produced leaflets in 1996 entitled *Before you Label People, Look at their Contents*, encouraging six steps to end stigma:

- Learn more
- Insist on accountable media
- Obey the laws in the ADA
- Recognise and appreciate the contributions to society made by people who have mental illness
- Treat people with the dignity and respect we all deserve
- Think about the person – the contents behind the label (SAMHSA 1996)

In 1998 SAMSHA, user/survivor and professional organisations 'walked the walk' for an awareness of mental illness in Washington, in what some activists affectionately dubbed the 'million mad march'.

All these initiatives have used methods deemed by research to be likely to be effective and have promoted new narratives: that user/survivors can contribute (not just take); that 'different' experiences – such as visions and voices – can be interesting (not

a

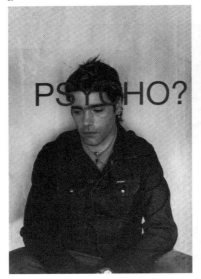

PEOPLE WITH
MENTAL HEALTH
PROBLEMS ARE
MORE LIKELY TO
BE ATTACKED
THAN THEY ARE
TO ATTACK
OTHERS.

WHY USE
LABELS WHEN
THEY DON'T FIT?

Jim isn't a 'psycho'. He is, however, unwell and finding it hard to cope.

He finds the kind of things most of us take for granted

like getting out and about and being active a real challenge.

But his nightmare really began a couple of months ago.

It started with name calling. Quiet by nature, Jim just looked at the floor.

Then the hitting started.

They could see he was defenceless. They knew he wouldn't fight back.

He didn't. He gets out of hospital next week.

Mind
The Mental
Health Charity

b

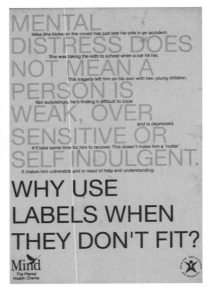

MENTAL
DISTRESS DOES
NOT MEAN A
PERSON IS
WEAK, OVER
SENSITIVE OR
SELF INDULGENT.

WHY USE
LABELS WHEN
THEY DON'T FIT?

Mike (the bloke on the cover) has just lost his wife in an accident.

She was taking the kids to school when a car hit her.

This tragedy left him on his own with two young children.

Not surprisingly, he's finding it difficult to cope

and is depressed.

It'll take some time for him to recover. This doesn't make him a 'nutter'.

It makes him vulnerable and in need of help and understanding.

Mind
The Mental
Health Charity

Figure 11.2   Health Education Authority/Mind postcards

frightening); that user/survivors' personal stories are engaging; and that user/survivors, far from just being the perpetrators of violence, are victims of violence and discrimination.

Around the world, considerable imagination has been used to create events to gain media attention. 1996 World Mental Health Day included celebrations with poetry and drama in Botswana, a parade with police band in Zimbabwe, the launch of a magazine edited by users in Romania and a meeting on women's mental health in Togo, where women first found the topic insulting but later demanded an additional session. Lessons have been drawn and conveyed worldwide, for example, on how marches and parades can 'draw in' passers-by (World Mental Health Day 1997).

There are also lessons to be learnt from the way in which the wider disability movement has made news, often combining direct action with sharply phrased slogans ('Piss on pity', 'Deaf president now', 'What good is the ADA if you can't even get out of bed in the morning?' and so on). They have become adept at mobilising activists fast. In 1991, a Los Angeles radio programme asserted that it was irresponsible for a mother to bring a child into the world with a 50% chance of disability. The disability community immediately made and distributed 100 copies of the tape to activists and media 'friends'. They devised three clear messages: that women with disabilities have a right to have children; that the radio show demonstrated eugenics thinking; and that a disability is not a disease. They generated considerable local and national media debate (Hartman and Johnson 1993).

Groups have acted to change, rather than just use, the media. They have met with editors, set up fellowships for journalists (the Carter Center), given awards for enlightened and terrible journalism, and held seminars in which editors and journalists educate and debate with each other. The latter can help to avoid the effect of resistance on the part of journalists to messages that they perceive as 'politically correct', didactic or driven by narrow sectional interests (Wahl 1995, Haller undated). In 1999 the American disability movement's efforts to engage editors in telling positive stories about the ADA bore fruit, with the publication of an article in the *Wall Street Journal* – previously a critic of the ADA – stating that the ADA had gained widespread support from the public and business, and had 'elevated the awareness of, and respect for, the millions of Americans with disabilities' (*Wall Street Journal*, 11 March, 1999).

Mental health groups have engaged with 'deliberative media' or 'public journalism', used first in relation to crime to spark public engagement (Hume 1995). A British citizens' jury on mental health policy found that, with evidence received over several days from local users, professionals and relatives, the public 'jury' became more supportive of non-institutional services and more aware that 'community care' could work (Institute for Public Policy Research 1996). Critics of these developments argue that they jeopardise the objectivity of reporting. Mental health reporting is already patently unbalanced: whatever two 'poles' of an argument may be chosen, they rarely include the user/survivor's perspective; often, they ignore the factual context entirely. But, given the high financial cost of citizens' juries, other interactive media need to be explored to enable the public to give full consideration to mental health issues – rather than just being scared by the latest homicide.

Targeting

Educational efforts can be directed at people with particular power in the lives of user/survivors – employers, judges, politicians – or at those with the most discriminatory attitudes – parents, older people, young men. Both strategies are important. It is critical to know current attitudes and build realistically upon them.

In practice, there has been little targeting of parents or older people. Young people are prioritised: they will form the next generation of parents and transmitters of values and their high suicide rates are viewed with more political concern than the (higher) suicide rates of older people. Supportive education for older people might, however, reduce the tremendous powerlessness of older user/survivors, both by making it easier for older users to voice concerns and by encouraging inclusion in older people's social networks.

Messages targeting parents need to be piloted through parenting groups and magazines, for example, the message that good parenting is about teaching children to respect people who are different, not keeping children away from user/survivors nor teaching them to be afraid.

Young people have been targeted through art, speech competitions and drama, for example the powerful *Cracked*, premiered at the Edinburgh Festival in 1997 to positive reviews and subsequently presented in schools and colleges, with accompanying interactive exercises: examining media imagery, designing posters, and deciding how the school can reduce stigma (Wellcome Trust 1997).

In the US, the Southern Poverty Law Center's Teaching Tolerance project gave students tasks such as writing an essay on 'What does it mean to be an American?' or imagining setting up a talk show on intolerance in America, explaining who would be invited to participate and why. This work looks at inclusion across many types of difference – religious, ethnic, sexual. Inserting mental health inclusion into such debates gives us a new framework, away from the usual emphasis on danger or, at best, the need to look after one's own mental health (Carnes 1995).

Education has been targeted by gender. The Health Education Authority/Mind project created a controversial card shaped like a dog's turd, with the slogan 'Feeling crap?', designed to encourage boys to talk. Pre-testing showed that boys found it funny and thought provoking. Those (older) people deciding whether to run it hesitated – but eventually agreed that effectiveness with the target audience was more important than their own aesthetic scruples.

For all these considerable efforts to grab people's attention with new narratives and to target effectively, discrimination in public debate remains rife; the mental health movement also has to 'respond'.

Challenging negative messages

Wahl (1995) notes that positive public education strategies find it hard to compete with 'the steady flow of polished and powerful media portrayals of individuals with mental illnesses as odd, evil and laughable'. User/survivor groups simply cannot afford advertising or significant media access.

There are a number of success stories – albeit few formal evaluations – that suggest lessons on how to challenge the media and product marketing. It can be useful to strike pre-emptively. The American National Stigma Clearing House found out that Superman was to be killed by a 'superlunatic' from an interplanetary insane asylum – and persuaded scriptwriters to have him die some other way.

A negative message can be turned in a new direction by advocates. In 1995, an inquiry into a homicide was published as a book entitled *The Falling Shadow*. Instead of just criticising its recommendation of more compulsory treatment – which would give its authors further opportunity to explain the violence making this 'necessary' – Kate Harrison of Mind argued that the title, *The Falling Shadow*, was reminiscent of a horror movie and that the cover illustration was melodramatic. This effectively hijacked the agenda, in the interests of user/survivors, by introducing a discussion of how mental illness is generally portrayed.

When adverts for the film *Crazy People* appeared in Philadelphia with the slogan 'Warning: crazy people are coming' and then 'Warning: crazy people are here', advocates picketed the cinema and the local newspaper, which had offered free tickets to all those who could prove that they were crazy. The outcome was a written apology from the newspaper, a cessation of the offensive adverts, and articles locally and nationally about the fracas, which highlighted the advocacy organisations' concerns.

This type of work requires tactical skill: to ride the waves of the narratives that are 'out there' in the public debate, to keep balance and to steer to the desired destination – only to duck and weave again as the pattern of comment and counter-comment continues.

Some groups have produced guidelines for journalists, for example, arguing 'journalists wouldn't get away with using words like nigger or queer – so don't call us psychos' (National Union of Journalists 1997). Advocates have used praise constructively and built relationships that have later led to more positive coverage.

The National Stigma Clearing House has had numerous successes in getting product advertising, or whole product lines, removed. When Daffy's (a clothes shop) ran an advertisement featuring a straitjacket to promote cut price clothing, pickets of stores were organised, complaints filed to the Human Rights Commission and protests made to advertising leaders (who had honoured the advertisement with an award). As a result, Daffy's scrapped the advert, providing local and national publicity, reprimands were issued by the Human Rights Commission, and key advertising leaders apologised.

The National Mental Health Association and others achieved the withdrawal of the 'psycho trainer' sports shoe. In Britain, East Suffolk Mind got the 'schizo pencil sharpener' withdrawn from a major supermarket: with a 'split personality', it didn't know 'what to sharpen'.

Co-ordination of complaint and constructive comment can be highly effective. The American National Stigma Clearing House puts out regular 'alerts' to 'stigma busters' across the country, thus enabling numerous people to influence the makers of film, media programmes or advertisements. The British Schizophrenia Media Agency supports user/survivors in speaking publicly of the impact of discriminatory images upon them.

Attempts at making formal complaints have met with mixed success. In 1996, Mental Health Media won a complaint against the British Press Complaints Commission. A man who was a user of mental health services had given Princess Diana a peck on the cheek – with her permission – although the permission did not stop a tabloid newspaper from reporting the incident in alarmist tones. In 1996, a nurse was struck off a professional register when he was found to have given confidential information about a Special Hospital patient to a tabloid newspaper. This has not, however, stopped further shocking staff breaches of patient confidentiality.

Organisations have issued booby awards. The American National Stigma Clearing House gave its House of Shame award to a promotion of Halloween Horror Nights at a Hollywood theme park, featuring a distressed man in a straitjacket. As Jean Arnold of the Clearing House put it, 'when corporate giants callously jeer people with disabilities to sell products, industry self-monitoring has clearly broken down' (press release, 8 December 1997).

Others have challenged charity fundraising. Corbett and Ralph note that charities, in competing for their market share, 'sell' disability by promoting either images of fear or 'a rosy glow, a feeling of inner good' for the giver. Both risk losing any vestiges of dignity and pride (Corbett and Ralph 1994). In the UK, SANE produced posters in the late 1980s featuring lurid images of people with mental health problems, with captions such as 'He thinks he's Jesus, you think he's a killer, they [the professionals] think he's fine.' The Advertising Standards Authority received a record number of complaints and the posters were withdrawn. In the 1990s, SANE's Chief Executive continued to be criticised for exaggerating violence; one article she wrote was headed 'Carnage in the Community'. For example:

> The fact that her words were published, that Ms Wallace is allowed to continue with her insinuations, is a reflection of the readiness of the media to use demonisation as a way of selling newspapers (Ramon 1996).

In 1997, the President of the British Royal College of Psychiatrists stated that a *Panorama* programme in which psychiatrists highlighted violence, to emphasise the need for resources, was unethical. The Chair of the NHS Trust featured, Professor Elaine Murphy, publicly apologised for the Trust's involvement in the programme and wrote to all service users expressing her apology, thus setting a standard for ethical practice.

Professionals have an obligation to develop a range of other compelling messages to attract resources, and not to engage in discriminatory public behaviour. Berlin and Malin (1991) note that an 'ivory tower' approach, rejecting all media work, can be problematic, although not as problematic as irresponsible comment.

User/survivors and allies need to convey a clear and convincing message about why they are objecting to particular stories. A simple general point – for example, that users want the chance to contribute to society – can be repeatedly inserted into objections to different negative stories. Clarity is needed on contentious issues. Take violence. Some organisations rely on the notion that 'users are no more violent than anyone else' (see, for example, Health Education Authority 1997b). This is not confirmed by research, which tends to suggest that active psychosis is linked to a raised risk of violence, albeit far less so than using drugs or alcohol (Sayce 1995a). Organisations denying this are likely to be disbelieved. And if they give evasive information to advocacy groups, they will find their supposed ammunition trumped by other players – psychiatrists familiar with the research literature, and journalists. A more promising approach is that adopted in the US by the National Stigma Clearing House, who, with the academic John Monahan, produced a consensus statement on violence and mental disorder. It combined accurate data with the strong message that user/survivors are responsible for a tiny fraction of violent crime.

We know that the belief that user/survivors are violent is associated with social distance (Link et al. 1992); reducing this fear is critical to social inclusion work. A number of messages need to be tested for effectiveness: that most crime is committed by people who are sane; that user/survivors often commit crimes for the same reasons as other people (poverty, drink and drugs, family/relationship frustrations); that it is extremely rare for user/survivors to attack someone they do not know; that user/survivors are more often victims than perpetrators; and – critically – that user/survivors can usually be held responsible. We also need to test whether such messages require interactive situations or whether they can have impact through the general mass media.

There is also a need to generate a more realistic public debate about risk than at present. It is impossible to predict every crime; we cannot have a completely risk-free society. Yet the public appears increasingly risk averse. In relation to the fear of crime, Fattah (1984) notes that the public does not understand that parole and probation involve calculated risks. They naïvely believe that shutting people in institutions stops risk – when in fact prison is 'a short term insurance policy and a dubious one at that'. The same is true of compulsory detention, supervision and treatment. These are hard messages to convey to a frightened public, yet the public does hold complex views of the patterns of risk in mental health, including the risk of users joining the 'underclass' or being disempowered by professionals (Ryan 1998). Establishing effective methods of building on this understanding is high priority.

Conclusion

We should not assume that 'educating' the public – informing them of the true incidence of mental health problems, or promoting the idea of a 'continuum', or explaining that the public's attitudes can make a difference – will act as a panacea. Many of these messages may be disbelieved or ignored as boring and irrelevant.

Nevertheless, there is an increasing body of research, and practice examples, that suggest a number of key success factors in shifting public discourse: starting from people's current beliefs, drawing out the positive strands and minimising the negative; emphasising users' contributions; having user/survivors – properly supported – or peers delivering the messages (backed by 'experts' when this is tactically indicated); and providing opportunities for interactive debate. Artistic approaches may provide an emotional, humorous or aesthetic counterbalance to the power of 'psycho-killer' imagery. In media work, the key is to be strategic – not only to complain about the negative, but also to set new narratives running and to steer old, negative stories off course.

We need to work with the people we are 'targeting', not to see them as passive recipients of our 'correct' messages, but to engage in dialogue. There are many messages that still require evaluation with particular groups, for example parents, who hold especially discriminatory attitudes but have been largely neglected by education initiatives.

We cannot assume, however, that even where we succeed in influencing attitudes – and even where this coincides with successes in changing law and policy – this will necessarily change behaviour. We also need to make inclusion happen, at the grassroots – to put enlightened policies, where they exist, into meaningful practice, and to capitalise on the research finding that public education is most effective where it combines educational messages with grassroots approaches that bring user/survivors into contact with different communities (Barker *et al.* 1993, Repper *et al.* 1997).

CHAPTER 12

Making Inclusion Happen at the Grassroots

Discrimination is overcome at the grassroots, not by writing policies in Washington (co-ordinator, user-run drop-in centre, 1995).

Laws and policies do not always change behaviour on the ground. The British Disabled Persons (Employment) Act 1944, requiring employers to employ a quota of 3% of disabled people, was never enforced; in 45 years, there was a sum total of 10 prosecutions, despite widespread non-compliance (Bynoe *et al.* 1991). Equally, some changes do not need policies: Aidan Shingler simply produced his art and exhibited it in Durham Cathedral (see Ch. 11). Most of the things that people 'just do' are, however, less visible. They happen locally. They are sometimes much aided by the legal framework or by a national public education campaign. But they are not adjuncts; they are core social inclusion activities.

The aim of inclusion is not a contradiction to creating user-only support and consciousness raising, but choosing safe users' space – anywhere from the local self-help group to the user-run hotel in Helsingborg (Sweden) – is very different from being with user/survivors because no one else will have you. The role of user-only space might even change if people could move in and out of the mainstream as they wished. The aim of inclusion is to ensure that people can join non-segregated life as and when they choose.

A powerful way to change public reaction to the idea of, for example, people diagnosed with schizophrenia working, is to do it. Once managers and workers have experience of working alongside someone who has chosen to be open about their diagnosis, prejudices tend to fall away. The most effective methods of influencing attitudes involve contact – preferably ongoing contact – between users and non-users, in a structured setting (as was shown in Ch. 11). Going to work is a structured and purposive activity; it enables, sometimes obliges, people to adapt their behaviour; it is likely to be at least as significant as specific educational projects in breaking down prejudice.

User groups working for social inclusion

The Charlottesville On Our Own user-run drop-in centre builds networks with people with multiple problems – people in the so-called 'underclass' – and provides a sense of community that people want to make use of. When I visited, the place was packed with people who support each other with all kinds of life problems. People may need food, help in getting food stamps, somewhere to sleep, de-tox if they want it, safety from violence and a chance to seek work. User/survivors make relationships with local shops and restaurants, some of whom donate food. The office voice mail can be used as a return telephone number by people who are homeless and seeking work.

User/survivors go out and train employers on the ADA and constantly negotiate for what individuals need with housing and welfare agencies. They visit people in jail and advocate on their behalf.

> Services are provided within the community, utilising natural supports: friends, family, community institutions. There are consumers who want their families to be an integral part of their lives, and request that we assist them in mediating differences. Others may wish to develop friendships with neighbors. We often attend social gatherings [with consumers]. In the past these members often remained isolated, their only social contacts were with other consumers or family. We encourage consumers to join clubs, attend concerts, and become active members of any and all groups and churches (Silverman 1997).

At the grassroots, projects like this or the Berkeley drop-in centre described in Chapter 8 exemplify what anti-discrimination work is all about.

First, they themselves aim not to discriminate. Unlike many professionally run day centres and clubhouses, they do not exclude people who have a criminal record or a drug problem. My conversations in these projects indicated a high proportion of people with serious mental health, alcohol and drug problems. They had successfully reached out to many people of colour and to openly gay people. Some were escaping from more structured and staff-dominated day-care environments where they felt less at ease. For example, one man who was unable to work with anyone with whom he felt paranoid, and who had been deemed unable to work, found that he could work in the drop-in centre.

Second, they aim to contribute to communities:

> We are good neighbours, offering assistance to others during inclement weather, by shovelling snow, if necessary. We are part of the landscape, and find that the more our neighbours get to know us, the more we are accepted as people, not mental patients (Silverman 1997).

Third, such centres model how workplaces could be made fully accessible to people with severe and fluctuating difficulties rather than just to people who are 'marginally disabled' (see Ch. 9). In the Berkeley Center, about a quarter of users are employed on a substitution basis. If someone is unwell, someone else fills in.

Fourth, they often engage in activism, which, according to Judi Chamberlin, 'goes to the heart of combating stigma, because it allows people you are dealing with, as well as the media and the general public, to see ex-patients as strong, articulate, active people, standing up for what they believe in' (Chamberlin, in Zinman *et al.* 1987).

Many user-run groups have moved from consciousness raising – sharing experiences of being in hospital, developing thinking and support on what the status of 'mental patient' means – through to running campaigns to protest against involuntary treatment or gain improved access to housing (Zinman, in Zinman *et al.* 1987). Coalitions with groups such as the Grey Panthers have achieved a number of goals, including ensuring that other marginalised groups – old people or refugees – have access to user-run services; enabling users to gain access to these other support systems; and raising awareness among potentially like-minded people, who may become allies later.

User-run services, which have attracted increasing energies, have struggled with a number of dilemmas. These include: discriminatory attitudes from some users, who feel that professional staff will inevitably be more trustworthy or knowledgeable; resistance from professionals; the need to challenge user-workers who begin to use power in ways that de-power other users; and the difficulty of jointly developing rules amidst fears that any rules may repeat the oppressive practices of some psychiatric services (Mowbray *et al.* 1997, Silverman 1997). Solutions have been proposed. Users have written rules: Howie the Harp produced guidelines on records, which state that user-run services should 'never ever' give out any information on individuals without written permission, and that user/survivors should be able to opt out of all or some record keeping if they wish (Zinman *et al.* 1987). Quality has been addressed through the independent user monitoring of user-run services (Joe Rogers, personal communication, 1997).

Evaluations show that user/survivors believe these services have a positive effect on their lives (Silverman 1997).

In Britain, user-run services have begun to develop, for example, in Woking, Lambeth and Sheffield. User organisations including Survivors Speak Out and UK Advocacy Network have produced charters for mainstream service providers and materials for user groups on effective advocacy.

Some groups have developed specific 'stigma-busting' projects. The STAR (STigma Awareness Research) project at the Club House in New Jersey involved a group of user/survivors sharing experiences of the impact of 'stigma' on their lives and developing problem solving on personal experiences in the social world. Users were trained to co-facilitate the project. One remarked:

> I always felt a lot of embarrassment. I had uncertainty about whether to disclose to people I knew, that I had schizophrenia. When I did, I talked with my family – and they are proud of me... I felt great.

The group invented role plays on issues like what to do when you bump into an old high school colleague at a bus stop and he or she asks, 'So what have you been up to?' – and then looks ready to run at the answer (being in a psychiatric hospital). The main emphasis is on awareness raising among users, a therapeutic and educational aim. This type of work needs to be complemented by initiatives designed to change discrimination in the external world.

Tackling discrimination within mental health services

Before mental health workers can operate fully as allies in anti-discrimination work, they need to overturn the discrimination that is virtually endemic within mental health services (see Ch. 3).

Some services have acknowledged the particular qualities that users can bring to mental health work, included the experience of mental health problems in all equal opportunities statements, advertised jobs as welcoming applications from user/survivors and provided support on the job for those requiring it – with positive results (Mowbray *et al.* 1997, Perkins *et al.* 1997). User/ survivors have begun to write positively of the transition from user to worker (see, for example, 'From schiz to shrink' by Carol North, in Mowbray *et al.* 1997).

These practices need extending. They may gradually encourage professionals to talk of user/survivors as equals – because users are now among them on staff. Staff also need training and support to make the shift. Mary Ann Beall told me that when she and another user started training in a Virginia state mental hospital, some staff 'came out' as users; some cried, others realised the depth of what had been wrong with the mental health system in which they worked.

In Maryland, a specific project, located at On Our Own, was designed to tackle stigma within the mental health services. By 1996, they had trained 600 people through 20 workshops for mixed groups of staff, user/survivors and family members. This enabled people to see issues from a number of different viewpoints, rather than discussions becoming polarised between staff and trainers, who could otherwise be perceived as 'stigma police'. Typical results were professionals realising that they had been handholding people too much, user/survivors understanding staff constraints and professionals exploring how their training had encouraged them to have an answer to every problem, which could create a miscommunication with user/survivors, who sometimes wanted simply to have someone to listen and be with them.

Fully non-discriminatory practice also requires a changed legal framework (see Ch. 1).

Social inclusion: the role of mental health services

Bates (1996), recognising that few long-term users of mental health services could name anyone they knew outside kinship and mental health service providers, set about turning mental health service delivery to the task of supporting user/survivors to gain access to a variety of local opportunities. They diverted some resources from day centres into workers who could make links with employers, colleges, sports facilities and art galleries, and who supported user/survivors in pursuing whatever they were interested in doing. Many obtained paid or voluntary work; over 100 gained mainstream college places. Word spread: 'Some users are not ready to venture out of the day centre but each one who does so comes back with a story and so everyone begins to contemplate change' (Bates 1996). Users and workers together delivered training to staff in job centres, volunteer placements, training agencies and museums in order to reduce discrimination.

Perkins and Repper (1996) have produced an overarching analysis of how clinical practice can be changed so that staff work 'alongside' people with long-term mental health problems, supporting them to gain access to communities of their choice. Clinical work is then planned according to user/survivors' goals. When user/survivors do not want to use mental health services, it is because they have found the services unacceptable. Therefore, 'the onus is on mental health workers and services to change what they do, rather than on the person to change their mind and accept what services think they need'.

The emphasis on user-defined goals changes the nature of assessment and outcome measurement. In the UK, user-designed assessment tools – such as Direct Power and Power Tools (Leader 1998) – began to enable some user/survivors to set their own goals, including ones in relation to experiences of discrimination. They might want support from a worker in responding to a family member who has made disparaging remarks about them, or in thinking through how they could meet a partner (often not easy; dating agencies, for example, often turn people away if they have a history of psychiatric treatment).

Discussions of clinical effectiveness are refocused towards the outcomes desired by users. It is not an effective intervention, for example, only to reduce symptoms, if the person's own main aim is to work out how to get a job, and the dose of medication needed to stop symptoms also reduces concentration, thus making work impossible. There is an urgent need to increase the evidence base in relation to user-defined outcomes and to measure success with individuals in relation to the outcomes that they most want.

When someone's goal is unlikely to be realised – perhaps because of discrimination – people appear to value acknowledgement of their aims and disappointments, and support to go some way towards the goal (Rogers and Pilgrim 1997). Professional attempts to steer people away from their goals can result in them feeling unheard.

Access to work and education

> Patients do not hold dances, they have dance therapy. They do not play
> volleyball, they have recreation therapy. They do not engage in group
> discussion, they have group therapy (O'Hagan, cited in Leibrich 1997).

In Chicago, rather than offering 'drama therapy', Thresholds rehabilitation programme negotiated with local theatres to establish job
placements (paid at minimum wage or above) in box office,
computer and administrative roles. Apprenticeships were established in lighting, make-up, music, set design, costume, acting and
direction. User/survivors 'encountered higher than average
acceptance from non-disabled co-workers, since theatre artists
appeared to be less fearful of persons with symptoms and impairments related to mental illness'. Thirty users completed apprenticeships, 10 in acting (Cook and Solomon 1993).

Many user/survivors simply need moral support to look for a
job; they need no particular accommodations. There are numerous
guides for user/survivors on how to survive at work (Mental
Health Law Project 1992, Canadian Mental Health Association,
undated); and for user/survivors and employers on reasonable
accommodations for those who need them (for example, Learning
Unlimited 1997; see also Ch. 8). Mental health workers can ensure
that users have access to this material.

Some people need more substantial support to get and maintain
work. Supporting people on the job is generally more effective than
step-wise preparation or skill development beforehand (Bond *et al.*
1997). Those providing the support can be other users (Mowbray *et
al.* 1997) or a variety of 'natural' supports, such as people within the
user's own network (Cook and Solomon 1993). Support for line
managers has been found to be crucial.

In negotiating supported employment, user/survivors and
workers need to be highly aware of what motivates employers. For
example, in one programme – a contract with an agency to comput-
erise personnel records – the contract manager told me that the
guarantee of a 'substitute' worker to cover illness was an important
motivator because it protected the company from risk. There were,
however, other factors. The minimum wage contract was less
expensive than in-house workers because of labour agreements.
The contract manager expected fewer complaints about rote work
from user-employees because of the opportunity it presented them.
The supported employment agency's support to line managers

was an important 'comfort factor'. Last, but by no means least, it fitted the company's desire to be seen as putting something back into the community; it could be presented at board meetings and in annual reports.

Employees in this programme did not appear to find the risk-protection arrangements patronising. They saw it, as the manager thought, as a big opportunity. They had all been hospitalised, in most cases repeatedly and/or for long periods: 'I've been trying to find a way to explain 15 years of unemployment.' Minimum wage is better than no wage. They also liked the fact it was long-term rather than the 6-month 'transitional' placement seen in many clubhouses.

People can sometimes move from supported to open employment, as managers become more confident and need less powerful 'comfort factors'. One man, in a different programme, obtained work as a clerk, with a job coach supporting him; he subsequently did not need the job coach and was promoted. His supervisor commented, 'at no point did employing Paulo put any of us out' (because the supported employment agency provided effective initial support to employee and manager). Mental health agencies are gradually building mutual understanding with employers. The level of support offered to users and managers needs to be calibrated according to their needs and confidence levels.

Similar knowledge is accumulating on supported education (Anthony and Unger 1991, Unger *et al.* 1991, Hooper 1996). User/survivors are beginning to be employed as supporters or 'mentors' to those attending college. Sharac *et al.* (1997) found that this benefited both students and mentors, and also influenced the local college's overall practices. Keys to success included the careful matching of student and mentor.

Mental health services are also just beginning to develop methods of supporting people in parenting (see Ch. 3).

Access to justice

User/survivors often have problems reporting crimes without having their diagnosis used to discredit them (as discussed in Ch. 3). In Wales, local Mind associations invited police to talk with users and staff, and involved them in workshops, which appeared to improve the police response to users' reports of crimes (Mind Cymru Council, personal communication 1997).

In the US, Hate Crimes legislation has been used as leverage. About 38 states had Hate Crimes Laws by 1997, although only a few – such as Oregon – covered disability. In Cook County, Illinois, the state's attorney's office appointed a disability specialist in the Victim-Witness unit. They produced a prosecutor's guide to hate crime, working closely for a year with African American, Jewish, gay, lesbian and disabled people. The resulting manual looked at hate crime as part of a continuing pattern of intolerance and promised a policy of aggressive prosecution. It advised how interviews with disabled victims should be carried out, for example, treating people as adults and not speaking through a companion. It proposed working with community advocates who could locate witnesses, provide emotional support to victims and give information to prosecutors.

Resulting work included outreach to communities at risk, training for police in the policy, and publicity. Despite this, victims with psychiatric disabilities still sometimes tended to drop cases when they realised what a court case would entail (see also Ch. 9). This kind of approach may, however, be extremely helpful in informing the public that disabled people are subject to intolerance and attack rather in the way in which black and gay people are. In the longer term, if court procedures can be made less impossibly daunting for user/survivors, prosecutions could also raise the awareness of user/survivors' vulnerability both among the general public and among user/survivors themselves, who might be less inclined to put up with abuse in the family, the institution and wherever it occurs.

In 1998 in the UK, a law was passed that introduced the specific criminal offence of racially motivated crime. Despite lobbying by gay activists, and discussion among disability groups, this was not extended to other hate crimes. Britain and other countries should examine carefully whether hate crimes law could be a useful step towards achieving justice for user/survivors; even without law, proactive work can be undertaken in partnership with the police and prosecutors to ensure that users are supported to give evidence and are taken seriously (Home Office 1998).

Organising services: networking for inclusion

In Britain, a number of primary health care settings have adopted methods of work that connect people with mental health problems into other opportunities. The Bromley by Bow Centre in East London offers linked services including health care, disability support groups, a nursery, women's groups, a café, Asian support groups, housing for homeless people – and support for people with serious mental health problems. User/survivors can access all the opportunities and get involved in systems advocacy on health and related issues (Callanan *et al.* 1997). For user/survivors, being actively included in primary care is in itself evidence of social inclusion, given evidence that people with serious mental health problems often experience low access to physical health care (Read and Baker 1996).

Other agencies – social services and voluntary organisations – also build links that can break down segregation. In Birmingham, a project initiated by a museum and supported by social services and health, offers opportunities for isolated Asian women, many with mental health problems, to get involved in tapestry in the local museum. The Act-up drama group in Dudley, supported by health staff, developed drama on mental health issues that was performed by users to professional and public audiences (Callanan *et al.* 1997).

Much of this work is achieved through partnerships. Health and social care workers need alliances that can deliver, for example, changes in the way in which social security staff treat user/ survivors, or an increased awareness in the local Chamber of Commerce. Sometimes a champion emerges from within one of these agencies: in California, a champion within the Rotary Club encouraged Rotary members to provide employment opportunities for user/survivors. Given a world-wide Rotary membership of 1.2 million, partnerships of this sort have strong potential.

Mental health workers can join existing coalitions – for urban regeneration, healthy cities and health promotion in schools (Ashton 1997) This can help ensure that others see the mental health links. For example, joint monitoring between education and mental health agencies might reveal that a reduced number of school exclusions could reduce later mental health problems (as well as the interlinked lack of opportunity and risk of crime), in which case, jointly planned 'inclusion' projects could be explored. They can ensure that user/survivors have a chance to join general projects aiming to counteract social exclusion. One example is the Circles Network in the UK, which assists people at risk of or experiencing social exclusion by helping them to build a circle of support, in effect an 'artificial' endeavour to create networks of friends where they have been destroyed or stunted because of disability, segregated services and other 'excluding' forces in people's lives.

Mental health workers can also add their voice of 'expert knowledge' to users' struggles for access, for instance by stating in court that a diagnosis of schizophrenia does not itself debar people from being good parents, thus potentially supporting individuals, as appropriate, and also educating judges.

It is a departure from traditional treatment models to aim to ease transitions for users – opening up new paths of access; increasing awareness in different communities; sharing knowledge with users and supporting them to extend their networks in the ways they want (rather than imposing inclusion as a new orthodoxy). It requires new training for many staff (Bates 1996).

The best defence against discrimination is to move forward positively to increase access. However, just as in media work, user/survivors and allies also need to nip opposition in the bud and, where it still occurs, to counter it effectively. Outright opposition can come from business, educational and other bodies reluctant to employ users or provide them with services. The battles are often lived out most publicly in opposition to user/survivors joining geographical communities.

Preventing and challenging 'nimby' campaigns

Research and lessons from experience of 'nimbyism' have reached certain consistent conclusions. This is best prevented through proactive community integration and education (Repper *et al.* 1997). While opposition can be extremely fierce, it almost always dies down once a project opens – and some of the most extreme opponents can become active supporters (Wahl 1993, Repper *et al.* 1997). Once opposition has started, small discussions, for example on neighbours' doorsteps, are useful (NHS Executive 1994). Public meetings are generally not helpful as they raise the temperature without providing opportunities to illuminate the issues (Scottish Association for Mental Health 1992, Repper *et al.* 1997).

An emphasis on discussions with neighbours does not mean overriding users' rights or giving neighbours a veto. Sayce and Willmot (1997), drawing on Repper *et al.*'s research, suggest two fundamental principles in 'anti-nimby' work:

1. Service users need opportunities, and support, to be as involved as they want to be in planning how to prevent and deal with community opposition. Having some control over the process can make it less distressing, and nothing overcomes the public's fear and prejudice quite as effectively as meeting individual service users where users want this to happen.

2. It is the right of service users to live in local communities and use mental health services, but working to build good relationships with local people can be constructive for everyone. If a service is obviously some kind of 'facility', local people are likely to be concerned. Sometimes their concern is helpful – they may question why a 'mini-institution' is being built and encourage a smaller service that actually suits users better. Often, the concern is hostile, in which case engaging with them is likely to avoid escalating opposition and build mutual understanding.

The first of these principles is often not followed. For example, Wolff *et al.*'s professionally run local education campaign – which found that contact between users and neighbours was more effective than the educational materials (see Ch. 11) – reached the conclusion that 'perhaps patients also need to be involved in discussion regarding their perception of their position in the community' (Wolff *et al.* 1996a). User/survivors need support, and acknowledgement, in relation to potential and actual opposition.

The second principle is also often breached, either by 'consulting' in ways that effectively capitulate to prejudice – as when a psychiatrist in Britain agreed to have a service open only on weekdays, when weekend opening had precisely been identified by user/survivors as their top priority – or by giving neighbours no information, which sometimes means intensified opposition from people who feel that they have been 'kept in the dark' (Repper *et al.* 1997).

Sayce and Willmot's (1997) suggestions for good practice are rooted in lessons learnt by 98 local non-profit organisations and a sample of NHS Trusts, national housing associations and voluntary organisations. Ideas include:

- being proactive in creating a positive understanding of mental health issues locally.
- being known in the community through anything from involvement in sports events and bric-a-brac sales to regular slots on the

radio – promoting positive messages, rather than waiting for a journalist's approach, which is usually framed within the existing discourse on violence.

- finding ways for user/survivors and the service to contribute to the community without expecting users to have to 'earn the right to live there' any more than anyone else.
- reducing local fear by providing a contact number that people can call if they have any concerns, and being available if they do.
- having facts and figures ready to dispel myths, for example, to show that house prices do not normally go down when mental health services open (Repper and Brooker 1996).
- involving user/survivors in discussions with neighbours if they wish or inviting neighbours to talk about general issues with user/survivors from another area, or with neighbours from another area who are no longer opposing a project.
- being prepared to listen to reasonable complaints from neighbours and make changes – for example, on facility size or parking arrangements – but not compromising on key service issues, such as having less than 24-hour staffing if this is what is needed.
- if it is user-run, selling the idea.
- never making promises that would lead to discriminatory exclusions, as in promising that there will be no one with a history of violence or a drug problem:

They want people using the facilities to have no history of drinking, taking drugs, committing crimes; to be paragons of virtue. How many of them could put their hands on their hearts and say they would fit those standards? (NHS Trust spokesperson).

If trouble persists, suggestions include:

- mobilising allies and political support.
- making use of the criminal law or disability discrimination law, if necessary, to prevent harassment, attack or exclusion.
- working with the police and media to reduce any escalation of opposition and marginalising those who remain obstinately bigoted, for example working with journalists to convey the fact that the majority of a neighbourhood is not opposed to the new service.

These strategies rely on having already built key relationships with journalists, the police, ally groups and local political leaders.

And finally:

Don't give up or apologise. People with mental health problems have a
right to live in the community.

Links between grassroots work and national activism

Sometimes local activism becomes national – and then influences
practice in numerous areas.

In 1996, Euan McGrory, a regional journalist, discovered that
patients in a psychiatric hospital had been buried in unmarked
graves. A carpenter who made coffins raised the issue: he wanted a
memorial created. McGrory ran a tireless campaign, achieving the
backing of the Prime Minister among others. Articles preached
dignity, and researched and recognised the lives of those who had
died. Money was raised, and a memorial was created, being dedi-
cated by a priest, who stated, 'In the 1970s... 60% of patients had no
visitors at all. The stigma of mental illness was so strong that a
convenient curtain was drawn over their lives. There was a front
page story in the *Northern Echo* and after that there was a huge movement in the community to befriend the patients.' These stories made
local people – the befrienders, priest and carpenter – into heroes who
created inclusion. In 1997, the government responded by issuing
guidance asking NHS Trusts to ensure that all patients have a proper
funeral in line with their beliefs, and a plaque or memorial.

In other cases, local and national work is planned together. Sayce
(1995a) documents how Mind's Stress on Women campaign
achieved some changes in national and local policy by combining
use of the mass media to build support, pressure on national
professional organisations, parliamentary lobbying, provision of
campaign packs and advice leaflets for users on how to complain,
so that local activists could influence service commissioners,
providers and politicians (see Ch. 7). National materials – arriving
simultaneously from government agencies, national professional
organisations and Mind – coupled with media profile, helped some
people locally to achieve influence: 'at last I don't feel I'm being
dismissed as "that feminist" for raising women's safety on the
wards', as one psychologist put it.

In the US, Internet lists have long been effectively used for the
targeted lobbying of key representatives on particular committees

and to alert activists to opportunities and equip them with research and practice data to inform lobbying arguments.

Locally, user/survivors and allies are aided in social inclusion work by legal frameworks and softer policy 'guidance'. Laws and policies, however, are only effective if they are 'grounded' in proposals emerging from the grassroots and in local testing. Often, more integrated policy is needed nationally, for example, between social security, housing and employment. It is local people who may have tried to build partnerships across agencies and who are best placed to identify the necessary changes in the policy framework. Evidence on effective campaigning methods suggests, as Shaw puts it, 'Don't respond, strategize'. The strategy must include maximum input from the grassroots.

The New Zealand Mental Health Commission laid out a strategic anti-discrimination framework in 1997. It analysed points of convergence with and difference from other minority groups, from people with AIDS to older people, and set objectives flowing from its research (see Ch. 11). It created a map of the 'journey' and clarified the individual responsibilities that could lead everyone to the destination. Goals included identifying and tackling discrimination in the mental health workforce, supporting Maori and Pacific Island people in dealing with discrimination, celebrating successful anti-discrimination work, taking cases of discrimination to the Human Rights Commission, equipping people to protect themselves against discrimination, improving media coverage, spreading stories of recovery, and strengthening consumer and self-help movements (Mental Health Commission 1997). The Commission built in feedback and evaluation. This approach fits the evidence accumulated in this book, that a single activity – such as law or education – is likely to be less powerful than strategies drawing on interconnected legal, public education and grassroots work.

In Britain, Mind ran a campaign from 1997, entitled 'Respect', with the strapline 'Time to end discrimination on mental health grounds' – in the public eye, in working life, as citizens. It combined lobbying, information for employers and prospective employees, individual test cases and proactive media work. It also drew on research into people's experiences of discrimination, including multiple discrimination, and built in evaluation and feedback.

In 1998, the World Psychiatric Association began piloting multistranded campaigns to counter discrimination on grounds of schizophrenia in a number of countries, beginning with Canada.

Conclusion

The transformation in mental health work envisaged by the aim of inclusion requires new skills in mental health workers, new respect for user/survivors as leaders in dismantling discrimination, and new negotiation and alliance building with people ranging from the police to disability activists, housing staff to political decision makers.

User-run projects are leaders in social inclusion work. Mainstream mental health services also play key roles – supporting user/survivors in access to employment and other opportunities, working proactively with user/survivors to prevent 'nimby' opposition, adding expert 'weight' to campaigns to break through discrimination, and modelling anti-discrimination practice. As long as mental health services continue to refuse user/survivors work on a wide scale, or treat them differently once employed; as long as disparaging attitudes pertain within services; as long as clinicians resort readily to compulsion rather than engage with people's own aims, professionals will be ill-placed to work as allies in social inclusion. Some mental health services are, however, changing – albeit at a varying pace. Some are employing 'out' user/survivors, introducing user-run training and promoting increased user power and social inclusion as mainstays of practice.

Action at local level makes the difference between laws and policies which are implemented and those which are ignored; it goes beyond laws and policies, into direct changes in attitudes and behaviour. At best, it feeds experience back into policy change nationally, even internationally, and informs public education work with evidence on which ideas have worked in changing the thinking in different communities. Those in direct contact with 'nimby' campaigners or schoolchildren may know exactly which messages do or do not work in encouraging increased respect for user/survivors.

This integration requires that user/survivors, allies and mental health workers push proactively for access to citizenship opportunities for user/survivors rather than waiting passively for rejections when they come, and that a 'movement' grows with strong links, and mutual learning, between those working locally, nationally and internationally, on policy and practice.

There is a growing knowledge base on how to achieve access to justice, education, employment and more. The challenge is to build effective partnerships to make it happen.

Conclusion

As the growing power of the user/survivor movement collides with pressures for increased social exclusion, we need robust, tested conceptual models to take the mental health world into a new phase of development. Otherwise, as cyclical analysts warn us (see Ch. 4), our latest idea will be just another in a long line of approaches – building asylums, closing them down again in favour of community care – that do not quite live up to their promise, if they take hold at all.

This book takes the view that this is not inevitable. The disability inclusion model can capitalise on a general recognition of the damage of social exclusion, and improve opportunities for user/survivors who are, at present, among the most excluded groups of all. This model, unlike others, does not contain within it traces of discriminatory thinking. It offers the potential to make a radical break from the 'unfinished history' of segregation (as described in Ch. 3). It combines an emphasis on the contributions that user/survivors make to society, with an attention to our collective responsibility to provide the access needed to enable that to happen. It expects user/survivors to take responsibility. It can be promoted as being fair for all.

To pursue this model means diverting some energies from old battles about whether 'mental illness' is caused by genes or social relations, whether solutions are primarily biochemical, emotional or spiritual, and turning them to concerted action to break down barriers and prejudice irrespective of the cause or remedy. Many user/survivors, relatives, friends and mental health workers could unite to improve citizenship opportunities. And while debate will rage over the discrimination inherent in mental health legislation (as we saw in Chs 4 and 6), significant achievements in employment or insurance would ultimately bring into radical question the way in which our laws subject people diagnosed as mentally ill to such coercive risk prevention measures, compared with other (sometimes far 'riskier') citizens.

An inclusion model involves working positively to build cross-disability support rather than waiting warily for other disability groups to address mental health issues more visibly. It means proposing overarching disability rights slogans that are mental health friendly – such as 'No to shame' rather than 'No pity' – and, reciprocally, making mental health groups and organisations accessible to people with a wide range of impairments. It means creating alliances with other excluded groups, from young people leaving care to asylum seekers. It also means taking positive steps to show employers, colleges and religious organisations that recruiting user/survivors can work: not only expecting inclusion but modelling, and explaining, how to do it.

To dismantle discrimination, one has to complexify issues. Most people have multiple identities: a woman user/survivor of Irish descent, a deaf person diagnosed with schizophrenia. Unpicking the interwoven stereotypes, understanding the way in which barriers compound each other, is central to inclusion work. Solutions, too, must be complex. It is no help to reduce employers' preconceptions if social security disincentives make work non-viable or if treatment regimes are premised on the notion that user/survivors will not work and that adverse drug effects such as thinking slowly or shuffling are therefore tolerable.

Evidence on anti-discrimination work is beginning to accumulate. We know that anti-discrimination law can begin to change the benchmark of what a society finds acceptable (see Ch. 8). While laws to regulate compulsory detention and treatment have been pursued far more vigorously than those to assure civil rights, or even entitlement to services, the international move to develop disability discrimination law, fuelled by nation-to-nation peer pressure and UN literature, is starting to shift the balance.

Yet while laws can change behaviours, they are also framed within, and can even entrench, prejudices that run deep in our culture. New law without new cultural ideas and images does not solve discrimination on its own.

Nor is the popular call for 'education' sufficient. Those who know more about mental health issues can be just as discriminatory as those who know less (Wolff et al. 1996b). Even where highly relevant education – delivered by someone trusted and combining the emotional power of art or stories with the best use of factual data – succeeds in altering attitudes, this does not necessarily change behaviour.

Direct contact between the public and user/survivors can be transformative:

> A few days after the first resident moved in, she was in the garden... when one of the neighbours came to the fence and started shouting abusively about her being allowed to live there. She said 'I'm terribly sorry my living here upsets you so much, but all I want to do is live here quietly and not be a nuisance to anyone'. The neighbour was like a pricked balloon! From then on everything changed and the same neighbour has been extremely supportive, even paying the vet's bill when a resident's cat was ill (Repper *et al.* 1997).

But such contact may require law, to enable the individuals to live next door in the first place. And contact on its own is no panacea. People may make an exception of the person they know – and still hold to the stereotype that mentally ill people generally are violent (Philo *et al.* 1993).

There is no single, logical line to follow from the intention to tackle discrimination to achieving change. All approaches are interdependent. We cannot start with attitudes and expect new behaviour to flow, nor leave it all to lawyers or journalists. But we can 'break in' to the current patterns of discrimination at different levels, with potentially dramatic cumulative results: through user/survivors meeting and consciousness raising, individuals taking risks in talking more widely about experiences of distress and discrimination – which means that contacts with users get generalised differently; through famous people 'coming out' and acting as role models, lawyers breaking new ground and gaining new judgements, advocates creating media stories that successfully compete with the 'psycho-killer' narrative, user/survivors supporting each other in 'recovery' and mental health workers supporting user/survivors to join the workforce or women's groups. And much more.

Research and practice examples show that this work is happening and can be highly effective. It needs to begin from where the neighbours, the employers, the TV watchers are, building on their positive views and practices, neutralising the negative. Approaches must be tested: exploring employers' priorities, evaluating messages to be used with different audiences. Adopting messages that only tell people that their current attitudes are wrong, or convey an idea that seems to them manifestly incredible, or ask them to do something that sounds impossible, is preaching in the wilderness.

Solid change happens when people connect with each other, pursue vigorous debate on concepts and methods, analyse why some approaches fail and share successes across different sectors and organisations – locally, nationally, internationally.

We are at an early point in the historical overthrow of discrimination against people diagnosed with a mental illness. It is all too easy at present for the public either to feel reassured at our progress – to remember that we no longer (usually) lock people up for life or tie them down – and/or to think that, really, people with mental health problems cannot be part of society. They should not be mistreated – but 'they' are not one of 'us'. The reality is that we are historically very near the eugenics movement. Mass forced sterilisation laws were only repealed 20 years ago, and the idea of worthy and unworthy lives is still in common currency. People do not have enough distance on this yet to see it for what it is. They therefore feel that change is impossible – or that it has already happened, at least as far as it needs to. The truth is that we have still not accorded value to people with mental health problems on anything like the same basis as other citizens; we still see them as 'undeserving'. This is a historical change in progress. How fast that change happens depends on the commitment and energies of people who want it to happen and on pooling our understanding of how to achieve it.

If inclusion becomes a major priority for mental health policy makers, practitioners and user/survivors, we could make the world a safer place for user/survivors, a place to feel established, to be 'insiders' without lying, to be included whether or not one is ever 'cured'. Work now to improve civil rights laws and to build new understandings may appear, in retrospect, to be a major step towards getting rid of films and press articles about 'psychos' and rates of employment among user/survivors of barely over 10%. One day, these may seem almost unbelievable pieces of historical barbarism.

References

ADA Summit (1990) President's Committee on Employment of People with Disabilities: Washington DC

Albee GW (1986) Advocates and Adversaries of Prevention. In Kessler M and Goldston ME (eds) *A Decade of Progress in Primary Prevention*. University Press of New England: Hanover

Albee GW (1992) Guest Speaker Presentation. In Trent DR and Reed C (eds) *Promotion of Mental Health*, Vol. 2. Avebury: Aldershot

Albee GW and Ryan K (1998) An Overview of Primary Prevention. *Journal of Mental Health*: **7**(5): 441–49

Albrecht G, Walker V and Levy J (1982) Social Distance from the Stigmatised. *Social Science and Medicine*, **16**: 1319–27

Allen M (1996) Separate and Unequal: The Struggle of Tenants with Mental Illness to Maintain Housing. *Clearinghouse Review*, November, 720–39

American Association of Pastoral Counsellors (1995) *Pastoral Counselling. A Ministry of Mental Health*. American Association of Pastoral Counsellors: Virginia

Anthony WA and Unger KV (1991) Supported Education: An Additional Program Resource for Young Adults with Long Term Mental Illness. *Community Mental Health Journal*, **27**(2): 145–56

Anthony WA, Rogers ES, Cohen M and Davies RR (1995) Relationships Between Psychiatric Symptomatology, Work Skills and Future Vocational Performance. *Psychiatric Services*, **46**(4): 353–7

Appelbaum PS and Grisso T (1995) The MacArthur Treatment Competence Study: 1. Mental Illness and Competence to Consent to Treatment. *Law and Human Behaviour*, **19**: 105–26

Asch A (1989) Reproductive Technology and Disability. In Cohen S and Taub N (eds) *Reproductive Laws for the 1990s*. Humana: Totowa, New Jersey

Ashton J (1997) *Concepts and Visions*. University of Liverpool: Liverpool

Audit Commission (1994) *Finding A Place*. Audit Commission: London

Awaz Group (1997) *Progress Report 1997*. Ethno Sensitive Mental Health Project: Manchester

Bair B (1982) 'The Full Light of This Dawn': Congressman John Fogarty and the Historical Cycle of Community Mental Health Policy in Rhode Island. *Rhode Island History*, **41**: 127–38

Baker P (1995) *The Voice Inside – A Patient's Guide to Coping with Hearing Voices*. Hearing Voices Network: Manchester

Barham P and Hayward R (1995) *Relocating Madness*. Free Association Books: London

Barker C, Pistrang N, Shapiro DA, Davies S and Shaw I (1993) You In Mind. A Preventive Mental Health Television Series. *British Journal of Clinical Psychology*, **32**(3): 281–93

Barnartt SN and Christiansen JB (1992) *Symbolic Visibility: The Deaf President Now Protest Four Years Later*. Paper to Society for Disability Studies Annual Meeting: Maryland

Barney K (1994) Limitations of the Critique of the Medical Model. *Journal of Mind and Behaviour*, **15**(1&2): 19–34

Bates P (1996) Lessons From Life. *Health Services Journal*, 3 October: 28

Bates P (1997) Paper to 'Challenging Perceptions' Conference: London

Bazelon Center for Mental Health Law (1997a) *Mental Health Consumers in the Workplace*; and Internet Updates. Bazelon Center for Mental Health Law: Washington DC

Bazelon Center for Mental Health Law (1997b) *People with Mental Disabilities and the Right to Adequate and Appropriate Public Services. Selected Case Law*; and Internet Updates. Bazelon Center for Mental Health Law: Washington DC

Beall MA (1995) Of Camels and the Eyes of the Needles: A Cautionary Tale. *Journal of the California Alliance for the Mentally Ill*, **6**(4): 51–2

Bedini LA (1991) Modern Day 'Freaks'? The Exploitation of People with Disabilities. *Therapeutic Rehabilitation Journal*, Fourth Quarter, 61–70

Benedek E (1995) *Beyond the Four Corners of the World. A Navajo Woman's Journey*. Alfred A Knopf: New York

Bennett NS, Lidz CW, Monahan J et al. (1993) Inclusion, Motivation and Good Faith: The Morality of Coercion in Mental Hospital Admission. *Behavioral Sciences and the Law*, **11**: 295–306

Bentall RP (ed.) (1990) *Re–constructing Schizophrenia*. Routledge: London

Benzeval M, Judge K and Whitehead M (1997) Tackling Inequalities in Health. In Sidell M, Jones L, Katz J and Peberdy A (eds) *Debates and Dilemmas in Promoting Health*. Open University/Macmillan: Basingstoke

Berkowitz ED (1996) Implications for Income Maintenance Policy. In West J (ed.) *Implementing the Americans with Disabilities Act*. Blackwell: Cambridge Massachusetts

Berlin FS and Malin HM (1991) Media Distortion of the Public's Perception of Recidivism and Psychiatric Rehabilitation. *American Journal of Psychiatry*, **148**(11): 1572–6

Berthoud R (1998) *Disability Benefits. A Review of the Issues and Options for Reform*. Rowntree: York

Beyond Reason (1997) *Art and Psychosis. Works from the Prinzhorn Collection*. Hayward Gallery: London

Bhugra D (1989) Attitudes Towards Mental Illness. A Review of the Literature. *Acta Psychiatrica Scandinavica*, **80**: 1–12

Blanch AK, Nicholson and Purcell J (1994) Parents with Severe Mental Illness and Their Children: The Need for Human Service Integration. *Journal of Mental Health Administration*, **21**(4): 388–96

Blanck PD (1994a) *Communicating the ADA. Transcending Compliance*. Washington Annenberg Program: Washington DC

Blanck PD (1994b) Employment Integration, Economic Opportunity and the Americans with Disabilities Act: Empirical Study from 1990–1993. *Iowa Law Review*, **79**(4): 853–924

Blaska B (1995) *Issues Regarding Mental Health Treatment of Adults Abused as Children. A Compendium from the Literature*. Prevail: Wisconsin

Bloch A (1997) Ethnic Inequality and Social Security Policy. In Walker A and Walker C (eds) *Britain Divided. The Growth of Social Exclusion in the 1980s and 1990s*. Child Poverty Action Group: London

Bogdan R and Taylor SJ (1989) Relationships with Severely Disabled People: The Social Construction of Humanness. *Social Problems*, **36**(2): 135–48

Bond GR, Drake RE, Mueser, KT and Becker DR (1997) An Update on Supported Employment for People with Severe Mental Illness. *Psychiatric Services*, **48**(3): 335–46

Boyd WD (1994) *A Preliminary Report on Homicide*. Steering Committee of the Confidential Inquiry into Homicides and Suicides by Mentally Ill People: London

Boyle M (1993) *Schizophrenia. A Scientific Delusion?* Routledge: London

Bragg M (1996) Out of My Mind with Terror. In Dunn S, Morrison B and Roberts M (eds) *Mind Readings. Writers' Journeys Through Mental States*. Minerva: London

Bray E (1998) *50:50. Welfare to Work for People with Disabilities and Long Term Health Problems*. E Bray: London

Breakey WR, Fischer PJ, Nestadt MD and Romanoski A (1992) Stigma and Stereotype: Homeless Mentally Ill Persons. In Fink PJ and Tasman A (ed.) *Stigma and Mental Illness*. American Psychiatric Press: Washington DC

Breggin P (1991) *Toxic Psychiatry*. St Martins Press: New York

Bright SB (1995) The Politics of Crime and the Death Penalty: Not 'Soft on Crime', but Hard on the Bill of Rights. *Saint Louis University Law Journal*, **39**(2): 479–503

Bright SB and Keenan PJ (1995) Judges and the Politics of Death: Deciding Between the Bill of Rights and the Next Election in Capital Cases. *Boston University Law Review*, **75**(3): 759–835

Bristol Crisis Service for Women (1994) *Understanding Self Injury*. Bristol Crisis Centre for Women: Bristol

Brockington IF, Hall P, Levings J and Murphy C (1993) The Community's Tolerance of the Mentally Ill. *British Journal of Psychiatry*, **162**: 93–9

Brooks L (1997) Dark Side of the Star. *Guardian*, 27 August, 2–3

Brown G and Harris T (1978) *Social Origins of Depression*. Tavistock: London

Bunting M (1996) Church that Ron Built. *Guardian*, 29 August, 2–3

Bureau B (1993) *On Using the Word Recovery Instead of Empowerment: Are we Being Courted or Seduced by the 12-Step Model?* National Empowerment Center: Lawrence, Massachusetts

Burkhauser RV and Daly M (1996) The Potential Impact on the Employment of People with Disabilities. In West J (ed.) *Implementing the Americans with Disabilities Act*. Blackwell: Cambridge, Massachusetts

Burns T (1997) TV Counselling. *Journal of Mental Health*, **6**(4): 381–7

Business Research Centre (1997a) Modifying the Community's Attitudes to People with Mental Illness. Pre-research prepared for John Boyd, Ministry of Health: Wellington, New Zealand

Business Research Centre (1997b) Public Knowledge of, and Attitudes to, Mental Health and Mental Illness. Research prepared for Ministry of Health: Wellington, New Zealand

Bynoe I, Oliver M and Barnes C (1991) *Equal Rights for Disabled People. The Case for a New Law.* Institute for Public Policy Research: London

Byrd K (1988) Theory Regarding Attitudes and How They May Relate to Media Portrayals of Disability. *Journal of Applied Rehabilitation Counselling,* **20**(4): 36–8

California Department of Mental Health (1989) The Well Being Project, Vol. 6. *Mental Health Clients Speak for Themselves.* Department of Mental Health, Sacramento

Callanan MM, Dunne TP, Morris DP and Stern RD (1997) *Primary Care, Serious Mental Illness and the Local Community: Developing a Commissioning Framework.* Salomons Centre: Tunbridge Wells

Campbell P (1996) The History of the User Movement in the United Kingdom. In Heller T, Reynolds J, Gomm R, Muston R and Pattison S (eds) *Mental Health Matters.* Macmillan/Open University: Basingstoke

Campbell T and Heginbotham C (1991) *Mental Illness, Prejudice, Discrimination and the Law.* Dartmouth: Aldershot

Canadian Mental Health Association (undated) *Strategies for Success: A Consumer's Guide to the Workplace.* Canadian Association for Mental Health: Toronto

Caplan PJ (1995) *They Say You're Crazy. How the World's Most Powerful Psychiatrists Decide Who's Normal.* Addison Wesley: Reading, Massachusetts

Carnes J (1995) *Us and Them: A History of Intolerance in America.* Southern Poverty Law Center: Montgomery, Alabama

Cassidy J (1997) The Next Big Thinker. *Independent on Sunday,* 7 December, 10–13

Center for Mental Health Services (1995) *Media Stereotypes of Mental Illnesses, their Role in Promoting Stigma, and Advocacy Efforts to Overcome such Stereotypes and Stigma.* Prepared by National Stigma Clearinghouse. Center for Mental Health Services: Maryland

Chadwick P (1997) *Schizophrenia: the Positive Perspective. In Search of Dignity for Schizophrenic People.* Routledge: London

Chamberlin J (1977) *On Our Own.* Mind: London

Chamberlin J (1993) Psychiatric Disabilities and the ADA. An Advocate's Perspective. In Gostin LO and Beyer HA (eds) *Implementing the Americans with Disabilities Act.* Brookes: Baltimore

Chamberlin J (1994) *Choice and Responsibility: Legal and Ethical Dilemmas in Serving Persons with Mental Disabilities.* National Empowerment Center: Lawrence, Massachusetts

Chamberlin J (1995) Psychiatric Survivors: Are We Part of the Disability Movement? *Disability Rag and ReSource,* March/April, 4–7

Chermayeff I, Wasserman F and Shapiro M (1991) *Ellis Island. An Illustrated History of the Immigrant Experience.* Macmillan: New York

Chomsky N, interviewed by Barsamian D (1994) *Secrets, Lies and Democracy.* Odonian Press: Tucson, Arizona

Citizens' Commission on Human Rights (1995) *Psychiatry. Eradicating Justice.* Citizens Commission on Human Rights: Los Angeles

Clare A (1977) *Psychiatry in Dissent.* Tavistock: London

Clarke AC (1997) *3001. The Final Odyssey.* HarperCollins: London

Clarke GN, Hawkins W, Murphy M, Sheeber LB, Lewinsohn PM and Seeley JR (1995) Targeted Prevention of Unipolar Depressive Disorder in an At-risk

Sample of High School Adolescents. *Journal of the American Academy of Child and Adolescent Psychiatry*, **34**: 312–21

Clore GL and Jeffery JM (1972) Emotional Role Playing, Attitude Change, and Attraction Towards a Disabled Person. *Journal of Personality and Social Psychology*, **23**: 105–11

Clough P and Lindsay G (1991) *Integration and the Support Service: Changing Roles in Special Education*. NFER-Nelson: Windsor

Cobb A (1993) *Safe and Effective? Mind's Views on Psychiatric Drugs, ECT and Psychosurgery*. Mind: London

Cobb A (1994) *Older Women and ECT*. Mind: London

Cogan J (1993) Accessing the Community Support Service Needs Women with Psychiatric Disabilities May Have Regarding Relationships. Doctoral Dissertation, Center for Community Change: Vermont

Connecticut Department of Health (1995) *Disclosure*. State of Connecticut Department of Mental Health and Addiction Services: Hartford, Connecticut

Convery P (1997) Unemployment. In Walker A and Walker C (eds) *Britain Divided*. Child Poverty Action Group: London

Cook JA and Solomon ML (1993) Thresholds Theater Arts Project: Final Report to the US Department of Education. Thresholds: Chicago

Corbett J and Ralph S (1994) Empowering Adults: the Changing Imagery of Charity Advertising. *Australian Disability Review*, June, 234–44

Corrigan PW and Penn D (1997) Disease and Discrimination: Two Paradigms that Describe Severe Mental Illness. *Journal of Mental Health*, **6**(4): 355–66

Coward R (1989) *The Whole Truth. The Myth of Alternative Health*. Faber & Faber: London

Crow L (1996) Including All of our Lives: Renewing the Social Model of Disability. In Morris J (ed.) *Encounters With Strangers. Feminism and Disability*. Women's Press: London

Cumming E and Cumming J (1957) Closed Ranks. An Experiment in Mental Health. Harvard University Press: Cambridge, Massachusetts

Dain N (1992) Madness and the Stigma of Sin in American Christianity. In Fink PJ and Tasman A (eds) *Stigma and Mental Illness*. American Psychiatric Press: Washington DC

D'Arcy C and Brockman J (1976) Changing Public Recognition of Psychiatric Symptoms? *Journal of Health and Social Behaviour*, **17**: 302–10

Darton K (1998a) History of Mental Health Factsheet. Mind: London

Darton K (1998b) Genetics Factsheet. Mind: London

Daughters of Utah Pioneers (1994) *Indian Tribes and the Utah Pioneers*. International Society Daughters of Utah Pioneers: Utah

Davis M (1992) *City of Quartz*. Vintage: New York

Davison C, Frankel F and Smith GD (1997) The Limits of Lifestyle: Reassessing Fatalism in the Popular Culture of Illness Prevention. In Sidell M, Jones L, Katz J and Peberdy A (eds) *Debates and Dilemmas in Promoting Health*. Open University/Macmillan: Basingstoke

Dear M (1992) Understanding and Overcoming the NIMBY Syndrome. *Journal of the American Planning Association*, **58**: 288–300

Deegan PE (1994a) Recovery: The Lived Experience of Rehabilitation. In Spaniol L and Koehler M (eds) *The Experience of Recovery*. Center for Psychiatric Rehabilitation: Boston

Deegan PE (1994b) The Independent Living Movement and People with Psychiatric Disabilities: Taking Back Control Over Our Own Lives. In International Association of Psycho-social Rehabilitation Services (ed.) *An Introduction to Psychiatric Rehabilitation*. IAPSRS: Maryland

Department for Education and Employment (1997) *Learning and Working Together for the Future*. DfEE: London

Department of Health (1993) *Omnibus Survey of Public Attitudes to Mental Illness*. Department of Health: London

Department of Health (1997) *Omnibus Survey of Public Attitudes to Mental Illness*. Department of Health: London

Disability Compliance Bulletin (1996) No ADA Violation in Parental Rights Case. *Disability Compliance Bulletin*, **6**(8): 11

Disability Discrimination Act (1995) Code of Practice for the Elimination of Discrimination in the Field of Employment against Disabled Persons or Persons who have had a Disability. The Stationery Office: London

Dobson F (1998) Department of Health Press Release, 29 July

Dole R (1994) Are We Keeping America's Promises to People with Disabilities? – Commentary on Blanck. *Iowa Law Review*, **79**(4): 925–35

Donnison D (1998) Sociology of Knowledge. *Prospect*, January: 11

Downie RS, Fyfe C and Tanahill A (1990) *Health Promotion: Models and Values*. Oxford University Press: Oxford

Dunn S, Morrison B and Roberts M (1996) *Mind Readings. Writers' Journeys through Mental States*. Mind/Minerva: London

Durlak JA (1998) Primary Prevention Mental Health Programmes for Children and Adolescents are Effective. *Journal of Mental Health*, **7**(5): 463–70

DVL Associates (1993) Attitude Research Conducted for the Central Office of Information. Central Office of Information: London

Employers' Forum on Disability (1996) *The Iceberg. Disabled People and Work*. Employers' Forum on Disability: London

Employers' Forum on Disability (1998) *Briefing Paper on Mental Health Difficulties*. Employers' Forum on Disability: London

Equal Employment Opportunity Commission (1992) *A Technical Assistance Manual on the Employment Provisions (Title 1) of the ADA*. EEOC: Washington DC

Equal Employment Opportunity Commission (1996) *Litigation of Cases under Title 1 of the ADA*. EEOC: Washington DC

Equal Employment Opportunity Commission (1997) *EEOC Enforcement Guidance: the Americans with Disabilities Act and People with Psychiatric Disabilities*. EEOC: Washington DC

Eru Pomare Maori Health Research Centre (1997a) De-stigmatisation Project. Pre-research with Pacific Island People. Prepared for John Boyd, Ministry of Health: Wellington, New Zealand

Eru Pomare Maori Health Research Centre (1997b) De-stigmatisation Project. Pre-research with Maori. Prepared for John Boyd, Ministry of Health: Wellington, New Zealand

European Day of Disabled Persons (1995) *Invisible Citizens. Disabled Persons' Status in the European Treaties*. European Day of Disabled Persons, Brussels

European Network of Users and Ex-users of Psychiatry (1994) *Mental Health and Disability*. European Network of Users and Ex-Users of Psychiatry: Brussels

European Newsletter of Users and Ex-users of Psychiatry (1995) **4**: 11

Evans JH (1976) Changing Attitudes Towards Disabled Persons. An Experimental Study. *Rehabilitation Counselling Bulletin*, **19**: 572–9

Faludi S (1991) *Backlash. The Undeclared War Against Women*. Chatto & Windus: London

Farina A, Fisher JD and Fischer EH (1992) Societal Factors in the Problems Faced by Deinstitutionalized Psychiatric Patients. In Fink PJ and Tasman A (eds) *Stigma and Mental Illness*. American Psychiatric Press: Washington DC

Fattah EA (1984) Public Opposition to Prison Alternatives and Community Corrections: A Strategy for Action. *Canadian Journal of Criminology*, **24**: 371–84

Faulkner A (1997) *Knowing Our Own Minds*. Mental Health Foundation: London

Faulkner A and Sayce L (1997) Disclosure. *OpenMind* **85**: 8–9

Favre G (1995) *Only Human: The New Biology of Our Genetics*. Sacramento Bee October 15: Sacramento, California

Feldblum CR (1996) The Employment Sector. Medical Inquiries, Reasonable Accommodation, and Health Insurance. In West J (ed.) *Implementing the Americans with Disabilities Act*. Blackwell: Cambridge, Massachusetts

Felner RD, Brand S, Adam AM *et al.* (1993) Restructuring the Ecology of the School as an Approach to Prevention during School Transitions: Longitudinal Follow-ups and Extensions of the School Transitional Environment Project (STEP). *Prevention in Human Services*, **10**: 103–36

Fisher D (1995) Disclosure, Discrimination and the ADA. *Journal of the California Alliance for the Mentally Ill*, **6**(4): 55

Foner J (1997) Poster: Ten Warning Signs of Normality. Support Coalition International: Portland, Oregon

Fonnebo V and Sorgard AJ (1995) The Norwegian Mental Health Campaign in 1992: Part 1. Population Penetration. *Health Education Research* **10**(3): 257–66

Foucault M (1967) *Madness and Civilisation. A History of Insanity in the Age of Reason*. Tavistock Publications: London

Frame J (1982) *To the Is-Land*. Paladin: London

Franklin D (1997) *Insuring Inequality: The Structural Transformation of the African American Family*. Oxford University Press: New York

Freedland J (1998) Out of the Bin and Glad to be Mad. *Guardian*, 21 January: 15

Freeman SA, Littlejohn SW and Barnett Pearce W (1992) Communication and Moral Conflict. *Western Journal of Communication*, **56**(Fall): 311–29

Gatherer A and Reid JJA (1963) *Public Attitudes and Mental Health Education*. Northamptonshire Mental Health Project: Northampton

Gerbner G (1990) Cited in National Stigma Clearing House, *Media Stereotypes of Mental Illness, Their Role in Promoting Stigma, and Advocacy Efforts To Overcome Such Stereotypes and Stigma*. US Department of Health and Human Services, Center for Mental Health Services: Maryland

Gifford G, Beresford P and Harrison C (1996) Further Links. *OpenMind* **78**: 20–1

Gillham JE, Reivich KJ, Jaycox LH and Seligman MEP (1995) Prevention of Depressive Symptoms in Schoolchildren: Two Year Follow Up. *Psychological Science*, **6**: 343–51

Gingrich N and Armey D (1994) *Restoring the Dream: The Bold New Plan by House Republicans*. Times Books: New York

Goffmann E (1961) *Asylums. Essays on the Social Situation of Mental Patients and Other Inmates*. Penguin: Harmondsworth

Goffmann E (1963) *Stigma: Some Notes on the Management of Spoiled Identity*. Penguin: Harmondsworth

Golden M (1991) Do the Disability Rights and Right-to-Life Movements Have Any Common Ground? *Disability Rag*, September/October : 1–5

Golding J (1997) *Without Prejudice. Mind Lesbian, Gay and Bisexual Mental Health Awareness Research*. Mind: London

Goldstein S (1997) Attention Deficit Hyperactivity Disorder. Implications for the Criminal Justice System. *FBI Law Enforcement Bulletin*, June, 11–16

Goleman D (1996) *Emotional Intelligence*. Bloomsbury: London

Gomm R (1996) Mental Health and Inequality. In Heller T, Reynolds J, Gomm R, Muston R and Pattison S (eds) *Mental Health Matters. A Reader*. Macmillan/Open University: Basingstoke

Gooding C (1994) *Disabling Laws, Enabling Acts. Disability Rights in Britain and America*. Pluto: London

Gooding C (1996) *Blackstone's Guide to the Disability Discrimination Act 1995*. Blackstone: London

Gostin LO (1993) Genetic Discrimination in Employment and Insurance. In Gostin LO and Beyer HA (eds) *Implementing the Americans with Disabilities Act*. Brookes: Baltimore

Gostin LO (1996) Litigation Review. In West J (ed.) *Implementing the Americans with Disabilities Act*. Blackwell: Cambridge, Massachusetts

Gould SJ (1985) *The Flamingo's Smile*. WW Norton: New York

Granger B, Baron RC and Robinson MCJ (1996) A National Study on Job Accommodations for People with Psychiatric Disabilities: Final Report. Matrix Research Institute: Philadelphia

Gray J (1992) *Men Are from Mars, Women Are from Venus*. Thorsons: London

Greenberg JS, Greenley JR and Benedict P (1994) Contributions of Persons with Serious Mental Illness to their Families. *Hospital and Community Psychiatry*, **45**(5): 474–80

Grisso T and Appelbaum MD (1995) *MacArthur Treatment Competence Study. Executive Summary*. MacArthur Foundation Research Network on Mental Health and the Law. University of Virginia: Charlottesville, Virginia

Grisso T and Appelbaum MD (1998) *Assessing Competence to Consent to Treatment: A Guide for Physicians and Other Health Professionals*. Oxford University Press: New York

Grobe J (ed.) (1995) *Beyond Bedlam. Contemporary Women Psychiatric Survivors Speak Out*. Third Side Press: Chicago

Gunnell D, Peters T, Kammerling R and Brooks J (1995) The Relation Between Parasuicide, Suicide and Psychiatric Admission and Socioeconomic Deprivation. *British Medical Journal*, **311**: 226–30

Hafer M and Narcus M (1979) Information and Attitudes Towards Disability. *Rehabilitation Counseling Bulletin*, **23**(2): 95–102

Haller B (undated) *The Social Construction of Disability: News Coverage of the Americans with Disabilities Act*. Penn State University: Middletown, Pennsylvania

Handy C (1994) *The Empty Raincoat. Making Sense of the Future*. Hutchinson: London

Hardman KLJ (1997) My Busy Mother. *Women and Mental Health Forum*, **2**: 8–9

Harris (1991) Public Attitudes Toward People with Disabilities. Survey conducted for National Organization on Disability

Harris (1994) Survey on Public Awareness of the ADA, quoted in Blanck PD (1994) Employment Integration, Economic Opportunity and the Americans with Disabilities Act: Empirical Study from 1990–1993. *Iowa Law Review*, **79**(4): 853–924

Harris (1995) Survey of Employment of People with Disabilities. Poll conducted for National Organization of Disability

Harris M (1994) *Magic in the Surgery. Counselling and the NHS. A Licensed State Friendship Service*. Social Affairs Unit: London

Harrison K (1998) Do We Need a Mental Health Act? *OpenMind*, **94**: 8–9

Hartman TS and Johnson M (1993) *Making News: How to Get News Coverage for Disability Rights Issues*. Advocado Press: Louisville, Kentucky

Hay LL (1996) *You Can Heal Your Life*. Eden Grove Editions: Middlesex

Hayward P and Bright JA (1997) Stigma and Mental Illness: A Review and Critique. *Journal of Mental Health*, **6**(4): 345–54

Health Education Authority (1997a) *Young People's Resources to Combat Stigma around Mental Health Issues. Qualitative Research to Evaluate Resource Materials*. HEA: London

Health Education Authority (1997b) *Making Headlines. Mental Health and the National Press*. Health Education Authority: London

Health Education Authority (1998) World Mental Health Day Pack

Henderson C, Thornicroft G and Glover G (1998) Inequalities in Mental Health. *British Journal of Psychiatry*, **173**: 105–9

Henderson M (1994) quoted in *Guardian*, 20 August

Heritage Foundation (1995) *Strangled by Red Tape. Collection of Regulatory Horror Stories*. Heritage Foundation: Washington DC

Herman JL (1994) *Trauma and Recovery*. Pandora: New York

Hills J (1998) *Income and Wealth: The Latest Evidence*. Joseph Rowntree Foundation: York

Home Office (1998) *Speaking Up for Justice. Report of the Inter-departmental Working Group on the Treatment of Vulnerable or Intimidated Witnesses in the Criminal Justice System*. Home Office: London

Hooper R (1996) Adult Education for Mental Health. A Study in Innovation and Partnership. *Adults Learning* **8**(3): 71–4

Hudgins EL (1995) Handicapping Freedom. The Americans with Disabilities Act. *Regulation*, **2**: 67–76

Hudson C (1993) Mental Health Policy in the US. In Kemp D (ed.) *International Handbook of Mental Health Policy*. Greenwood: Westport, Connecticut

Hume E (1995) *Tabloids, Talk Radio, and the Future of News: Technology's Impact on Journalism*. The Annenberg Washington Program, Communications Policy Studies, Northwestern University: Washington DC

Hutton W (1997) *The State To Come*. Vintage: London

Huxley P (1993) Location and Stigma: A Survey of Community Attitudes to Mental Illness: Part 1. Enlightenment and Stigma. *Journal of Mental Health*, **2**(7): 73–80

Huxley PJ, Raval H, Korer J and Jacob C (1989) Psychiatric Morbidity in the Clients of Social Workers. *Psychological Medicine*, **19**: 187–97

ICM (1990) Opinion Poll for Guardian Newspaper and National Schizophrenia Fellowship. NSF: London

Institute for Public Policy Research (1996) Citizens' Jury. Kensington, Chelsea and Westminster. 'People with Mental Illness Live in the Community: What Can Be Done To Improve the Quality of Life for Mental Health Service Users, Carers and their Neighbours?' IPPR: London

Jahoda M (1979) The Impact of Unemployment in the 1930s and the 1970s. *Bulletin of the British Psychological Society*, **32**: 309–14

Jamison KR (1995) *An Unquiet Mind. A Memoir of Moods and Madness*. Alfred A Knopf: New York

Jamison KR (1998) *Mood Disorders and Creativity*. Paper to Royal Festival Hall: London

Jenkins R (1997) Nations for Mental Health. *Social Psychiatry and Epidemiology*, 32

Jennings A (1994) On Being Invisible in the Mental Health System. *Journal of Mental Health Administration*, **21**(4): 374–87

Joffe H (1996) Aids Research and Prevention. A Social Representational Approach. *British Journal of Medical Psychology*, **69**: 169–90

Jones K (1960) *Mental Health and Social Policy 1845–1959*. Routledge & Kegan Paul: London

Jones L and Cochrane R (1981) Stereotypes of Mental Illness: A Test of the Labelling Hypothesis. *International Journal of Social Psychiatry*, **27**: 99–107

Katz P (1995) *The New Urbanism. Towards an Architecture of Community*. McGraw Hill: New York

Kemp D (ed.) (1993) *International Handbook on Mental Health Policy*. Greenwood: Westport, Connecticut

Kennedy M (1996) Paper to International Conference on Violence Against Women: Brighton

Kitzinger C and Perkins RE (1993) *Changing Our Minds: Lesbian Feminism and Psychology*. New York University Press: New York

Kitzinger J (1996) Media Representations of Sexual Abuse Risks. *Child Abuse Review*, **5**: 319–33

Koyanagi C (1995) *Turning the Corner. New Ways to Integrate Mental Health and Substance Abuse in Health Care Policy*. Bazelon Center for Mental Health Law: Washington DC

Kozol J (1995) The Kids That Society Forgot. *Washington Post*, 1 October

Kraus JF, Blander B and McArthur DL (1995) Incidence, Risk Factors and Prevention Strategies for Work-related Assault Injuries. *Annual Review of Public Health*, **16**: 355–79

Labour Force Survey 1997/8. In Department for Education and Employment (1998) *Unemployment and Activity Rates for People of Working Age*. Background Paper for Welfare to Work Seminar. DfEE: London

Laing RD (1960) *The Divided Self*. Tavistock: London

Lange JI (1990) Refusal To Compromise: The Case of Earth First! *Western Journal of Speech Communication*, **54**(Fall): 473–94

La Polla SM (1995) Disclosure. *Journal of the California Alliance for the Mentally Ill*, **6**(4): 53–4

Lattimer M (1994) *The Campaigning Handbook*. Directory of Social Change: London

Leader A (1998) *Power Tools*. Pavilion Publishing: Sussex

Learning Unlimited Limited (1997) *Put Your Company in Clover*. Mental Health Employment Promotion Training Kit. Learning Unlimited: Wellington, New Zealand

Leff J, Trieman N and Gooch C (1996) Teams Assessment of Psychiatric Services (TAPS) Project 33: Prospective Follow-Up Study of Long-Stay Patients Discharged from Two Psychiatric Hospitals. *American Journal of Psychiatry*, **153**(10): 1318–24

Leibrich J (1997) The Doors of Perception. *Australian and New Zealand Journal of Psychiatry*, **31**: 36–45

Levey S and Howells K (1995) Dangerousness, Unpredictability and the Fear of People with Schizophrenia. *Journal of Forensic Psychiatry*, **6**(1): 19–39

Levine M and Levine A (1970) *A Social History of Helping Services: Clinic, Court, School and Community*. Appleton-Century-Crofts: New York

Lindow V (1996) What We Want from Community Psychiatric Nurses. In Read J and Reynolds J (eds) *Speaking Our Minds. An Anthology of Personal Experiences of Mental Distress and its Consequences*. Open University/Macmillan: Basingstoke

Link BG, Cullen FT, Mirotznik J and Struening E (1992) The Consequences of Stigma for Persons with Mental Illness: Evidence from the Social Sciences. In Fink PJ and Tasman A (ed.) *Stigma and Mental Illness*. American Psychiatric Press: Washington DC

Link BG, Struening EL, Rahav M, Phelan JC and Nuttbrock L (1997) On Stigma and its Consequences: Evidence from a Longitudinal Study of Men with Dual Diagnoses of Mental Illness and Substance Abuse. *Journal of Health and Social Behaviour*, **38**: 177–90

Lister R (1997) From Fractured Britain to One Nation? The Policy Options for Welfare Reform. *Renewal*, **5**(3/4): 11–23

Littauer F (1986) *How to Beat the Blahs: Facing Depression with Courage*. Harvest Pocket Books: Eugene, Oregon

Livneh H (1982) On the Origins of Negative Attitudes Toward People with Disabilities. *Rehabilitation Literature* **43**(11–12): 338–47

Lombardo P (1983) Involuntary Sterilisation in Virginia: from Buck v. Bell to Poe v. Lynchburg. *Developments in Mental Health Law*, **3**(3): 17–21

Lombardo P (1985) Three Generations, No Imbeciles: New Light on Buck v. Bell. New York *University Law Review*, **60**(1): 30–62

Macaskill A, Macaskill N and Nicol A (1997) The Defeat Depression Campaign. A Mid-point Evaluation of its Impact on General Practitioners. *Psychiatric Bulletin*, **21**: 148–50

McCord C and Freeman HC (1990) Excess Mortality in Harlem. *New England Journal of Medicine*, **322**: 173–7

McGuffin P, Owen MJ and Farmer AE (1995) Genetic Basis of Schizophrenia. *Lancet*, 346, 9 September, 678–82

McNamara J (1996) Out of Order. Madness is a Feminist and a Disability Issue. In Morris J (ed.) *Encounters with Strangers*. Women's Press: London

McNeil JM (1993) *Americans with Disabilities 1991–2*. US Department of Commerce, Bureau of the Census: Washington DC

Maitland S (1997) Religion and Mental Health. Paper to Mind Annual Conference: Scarborough

Mancuso LL (1993) *Case Studies on Reasonable Accommodation for Workers with Psychiatric Disabilities.* Center for Mental Health Services and California Department of Mental Health: San Francisco

Mancuso LL (1996) *Roundtable on the Americans with Disabilities Act.* Center for Mental Health Services: Maryland

Masson J (1988) *Against Therapy.* William Collins: Glasgow

Matrix Research Institute (1995) *The Facts About Mental Illness and Work.* Matrix Research Institute and University of Pennsylvania: Philadelphia

Mayer A and Barry DD (1992) Working with the Media to De-stigmatise Mental Illness. *Hospital and Community Psychiatry* **43**: 77–8

Mental Health Association of Hong Kong (1993) *Annual Report 1992–3.* Mental Health Association of Hong Kong: Hong Kong

Mental Health Commission (1997) Discrimination Against People with Experiences of Mental Illness. Discussion Paper for the Mental Health Commission: Wellington, New Zealand

Mental Health Law Project (1992) *Mental Health Consumers in the Workplace. An ADA Handbook.* Mental Health Law Project: Washington DC

Metropolitan Washington Council of Governments (1995) *Mental and Substance Use Disorders: the Treatment of Dual Diagnosis. A Policy Report.* Metropolitan Washington Council of Governments: Washington DC

Miller LJ (1992) Comprehensive Care of Pregnant Mentally Ill Women. *Journal of Mental Health Administration,* **19**(2): 170–7

Miller PS (1995) Presentation to Department of Health and Human Services: Washington DC

Mind (1993) *Policy on Social Security.* Mind: London

Mind (1997a) Respect: Time to End Discrimination on Mental Health Grounds. Campaign Briefing. Mind: London

Mind (1997b) *Respect in Working Life.* Mind: London

Modood T, Berthoud R, Lakey J et al. (1997) *Ethnic Minorities in Britain. Diversity and Disadvantage.* Policy Studies Institute: London

Mollica RF (1983) The Threatened Disintegration of Public Psychiatry. *New England Journal of Medicine,* **30**: 367–73

Monahan J (1993) *Limiting Therapist Exposure to Tarasoff Liability. Guidelines for Risk Containment.* American Psychological Association: Washington, DC

Monahan J, Hoge SK, Lidz CW et al. (1995) Coercion to Inpatient Treatment: Initial Results and Implications for Assertive Treatment in the Community. In Dennis D and Monahan J (eds) *Coercion and Aggressive Community Treatment: a New Frontier in Mental Health Law.* Plenum: New York

Mori (1997) Attitudes Towards Schizophrenia. Research Study Conducted for Fleischman Hillard & Lilly

Morris J (ed.) (1996) *Encounters with Strangers: Feminism and Disability.* Women's Press: London

Mosher LR and Burti L (1989) *Community Mental Health: Principles and Practice.* Norton: New York

Moss K (1991) Lessons Learnt about Employment Rights of People with Mental Disabilities. *Policy in Perspective,* November/December: 1–5

Mowbray CT and Benedek EP (1990) *Women's Mental Health Research Agenda: Services and Treatments of Mental Disorders in Women.* US Dept of Health and Human Services, Occasional Paper

Mowbray CT, Moxley DP, Jasper CA and Howell LL (eds) (1997) *Consumers as Providers in Psychiatric Rehabilitation*. International Association of Psychosocial Rehabilitation Services: Columbia, Maryland

Mowbray CT, Oyersman D, Zemencuk JK and Ross SR (1995) Motherhood for Women with Serious Mental Illness. *American Journal of Orthopsychiatry*, **65**(1): 21–38

Moxley DP and Mowbray CT (1997) Consumers as Providers: Forces and Factors Legitimizing Role Innovation in Psychiatric Rehabilitation. In Mowbray CT, Moxley DP, Jasper CA and Howell LL (eds) *Consumers as Providers in Psychiatric Rehabilitation*. International Association of Psychosocial Rehabilitation Services: Columbia, Maryland

Muijen M (1997) Paper to Sainsbury Centre Conference: London

Muijen M, Marks I, Connolly J and Audini B (1992) Home-based Care and Standard Hospital Care for Patients with Severe Mental Illness: A Randomised Controlled Trial. *British Medical Journal*, **304**: 749–54

Mullen P, Walton VA, Roman-Clarkson SE and Herbison GP (1988) The Impact of Sexual and Physical Abuse on Women's Mental Health. *Lancet*, 16 April, 841–4

Mullen P, Wallace C, Burgess P, Palmer S, Ruschena D and Browne C (1998) Serious Criminal Offending and Mental Disorder: Case Linkage Study. *British Journal of Psychiatry*, **172**: 477–84

Murphy E (1991) *After the Asylum*. Faber: London

Murray C and Hernstein RJ (1996) *The Bell Curve*. Scribners: New York

National Academy of Social Insurance (1996) *Balancing Security and Opportunity: The Challenge of Disability Income Policy*. National Academy of Social Insurance: Washington DC

National Alliance for the Mentally Ill (1996) Open Your Mind. Campaign Pack, Survey and Insurance Briefings. NAMI: Washington DC

National Disability Council (1996) Opinion Leaders' Research Conducted for National Disability Council: London

National Institute of Mental Health (1994) *Primary Prevention in Mental Health: An Annotated Bibliography 1983–1991*. National Institute of Mental Health: Maryland

National Union of Journalists (1997) *Shock Treatment. A Guide to Better Mental Health Reporting*. National Union of Journalists: London.

Ndlovu V (1997) Current Status of Psychiatric Services in Matabeleland, South Zimbabwe. Unpublished paper: Zimbabwe

Nelson GD and Barbaro MB (1985) *Fighting Stigma: A Unique Approach to Marketing Mental Health*. Marketing Strategies for Human and Social Service Agencies. SERCO: Dayton, Ohio

Nergard J (1997) The Saami Concept of Psychosis. Paper to the International Conference on the Psychotherapy of Psychosis: London

New Zealand Ministry of Health (1997) *Mental Health Promotion for Younger and Older Adults. The Public Health Issues*. Ministry of Health: Wellington, New Zealand

NHS Executive (1994) *Dealing with the Nimby Syndrome*. 17: 2

NHS Executive (1996) *NHS Psychotherapy Services in England. Review of Strategic Policy*. NHS Executive: London

O'Donoghue D (1994) *Breaking Down Barriers. The Stigma of Mental Illness: A User's Point of View*. US, the All Wales User Network: Aberystwyth

Office of Technology Assessment (1994) *Psychiatric Disabilities, Employment and the Americans with Disabilities Act.* Office of Technology Assessment: Washington DC

Oliver M (1990) *The Politics of Disablement.* Macmillan: Basingstoke

Olsen F (1991) Statutory Rape: a Feminist Critique of Rights Analysis. In Bartlett KT and Kennedy R (eds) *Feminist Legal Theory.* Westview Press: Boulder, Colorado

Page S (1977) Effects of the Mental Illness Label in Attempts to Obtain Accommodation. *Canadian Journal of Behavioral Sciences,* **9**: 85–90

Palmer RL, Chaloner DA and Oppenheimer R (1992) Childhood Sexual Experiences with Adults Reported by Female Psychiatric Patients. *British Journal of Psychiatry,* **160**: 261–5

Parens E (1996) Taking Behavioural Genetics Seriously. *Hastings Center Report* **26**:(4): 13–18

Peck E and Barker I (1997) *Making Progress in Mental Health: A National Framework for Local Action.* King's Fund: London

Peck J (1996) Workfare. A Geo-political Etymology. Harkness Fellowship Report: Manchester

Pedro-Carroll JL and Cowen EL (1985) The Children of Divorce Intervention Program: An Investigation of the Efficacy of a School Based Prevention Program. *Journal of Consulting and Clinical Psychology,* **53**(5): 603–11

Pembroke L (1995) National Self Harm Network. *OpenMind,* **73**: 13

Perez C (1994) Peer or Mutual Self-Help in an Hispanic Culture Environment. In Harp HT and Zinman S (eds) *Reaching Across: II. Maintaining Our Roots/ The Challenge of Growth.* California Network of Mental Health Clients: Sacramento, California

Perkins R (1992) Catherine Is Having a Baby. *Feminism and Psychology,* **2**: 56–7

Perkins R, Nadirshaw Z, Copperman J and Andrews C (eds) (1996) *Women in Context.* Good Practices in Mental Health: London

Perkins RE and Foyster L (eds) (1997) Newsletter of the Women and Mental Health Forum, 2

Perkins RE and Repper JM (1996) *Working Alongside People with Long Term Mental Health Problems.* Chapman & Hall: London

Perkins RE and Repper J (1998) *Dilemmas in Community Mental Health Practice.* Radcliffe Medical Press: Abingdon

Perkins RE and Silver E (1994) Report of the Wandsworth Mental Health Needs Assessment Project. Pathfinder NHS Trust: London

Perkins RE, Buckfield R and Choy D (1997) Access to Employment: A Supported Employment Project to Enable Mental Health Service Users to Obtain Jobs Within Mental Health Teams. *Journal of Mental Health,* **6**(3): 307–18

Perlin ML (1995) Sanism and the ADA: Thinking about Attitudes. *Journal of the California Alliance of the Mentally Ill,* **6**(4): 10–11

Peters J (1997) Stigma and Discrimination against People who Have a Mental Illness: Mental Health Organisations' Views – a Survey Summary. Waitemata Health: Auckland, New Zealand

Pfeiffer D (1994) Eugenics and Disability Discrimination. *Disability and Society,* **9**(4): 481–99

Philo G, Henderson L and McLaughlin G (1993) Mass Media Representation of Mental Health/Illness. Report for Health Education Board for Scotland: Glasgow University

Pilgrim D (1997) *Psychotherapy and Society.* Sage: London

Pilgrim D and Rogers A (1993) *A Sociology of Mental Health and Illness.* Open University Press: Buckingham

Plumb A (1994) *Distress or Disability? A Discussion Document.* GMCDP Publications: London

Pointon A and Davies C (1997) *Framed: Interrogating Disability in the Media.* British Film Institute: London

Porter R (ed.) (1991) *The Faber Book of Madness.* Faber & Faber: London

Pozner A, Ng Mee Ling, Hammond J and Shepherd G (1996) *Working It Out – Creating Work Opportunities for People with Mental Health Problems.* Pavilion/Sainsbury Centre for Mental Health/Outset: London

Price J (1994) *The History of my Mental Illness.* Unpublished paper. Washington DC

Putnam RD (1996) The Strange Disappearance of Civic America. *American Prospect,* **24**: 34–48

Ralph S (1989) Using Videotape in the Modification of Attitudes Towards People with Physical Disabilities. *Journal of the Multihandicapped Person,* **2**(4): 327–36

Ramon S (1996) *Mental Health in Europe.* Macmillan: Basingstoke

Rapier J, Adelson R, Carey R and Croke K (1972) Changes in Children's Attitudes Toward the Physically Handicapped. *Exceptional Children,* **39**: 219–23

Read J and Baker S (1996) *Not Just Sticks and Stones. A Survey of the Stigma, Taboos and Discrimination Experienced by People with Mental Health Problems.* Mind: London

Read J and Campbell P (1995) *Workshop on Positive Aspects of Madness.* Mind Annual Conference: Blackpool

Read J and Reynolds (1996) (eds) *Speaking Our Minds: An Anthology.* Open University/Macmillan: Basingstoke

Re-evaluation Counseling Communities (1991) *What's Wrong with the 'Mental Health' System and What Can Be Done about it? A Draft Policy.* Rational Island Publishers: Seattle

Report of the Confidential Inquiry into Homicides and Suicides of Mentally Ill People (1996). Royal College of Psychiatrists: London

Repper J and Brooker C (1996) *A Review of Public Attitudes Towards Mental Health Facilities in the Community.* Sheffield Centre for Health and Related Research: Sheffield

Repper J, Sayce L, Strong S, Willmot J and Haines M (1997) Tall Stories from the Back Yard. A Survey of Nimby Opposition to Community Mental Health Facilities Experienced by Key Service Providers in England and Wales. Mind: London

Reynolds I and Hoult JE (1984) The Relatives of the Mentally Ill: A Comparative Trial of Community-oriented and Hospital-oriented Psychiatric Care. *Journal of Nervous and Mental Disease,* **172**: 480–9

Robert Wood Johnson Foundation (1990) *Public Attitudes Toward People with Chronic Mental Illness.* Robert Wood Johnson Foundation: New York

Rochefort DA (1988) Policymaking Cycles in Mental Health: Critical Examination of a Conceptual Model. *Journal of Health Politics, Policy and Law*, **13**(1): 129–52

Rodgers B (1990) Adult Affective Disorder and Early Environment. *British Journal of Psychiatry*, **157**: 539–50

Rogers A and Pilgrim D (1997) The Contribution of Lay Knowledge to the Understanding and Promotion of Mental Health. *Journal of Mental Health*, **6**(1): 23–35

Rogers A, Pilgrim D and Lacey R (1993) *Experiencing Psychiatry*. Mind/Macmillan: London

Rogers R (1997) *Cities for a Small Planet*. Faber & Faber: London

Rose D (1996) *Living in the Community*. Sainsbury Centre for Mental Health: London

Rosenbaum R (1990) Travels with Dr. Death, *Vanity Fair*, May, 206–37

Royal Pharmaceutical Society of Great Britain (1997) *From Compliance to Concordance. Achieving Shared Goals in Medicine Taking*. Royal Pharmaceutical Society of Great Britain: London

Rubenstein L (1996) People with Psychiatric Disabilities. In West J (ed.) *Implementing the Americans with Disabilities Act*. Blackwell: Cambridge Massachusetts

Rubenstein LS (1993) Mental Disorder and the ADA. In Gostin LO and Beyer HA (eds) *Implementing the Americans with Disabilities Act*. Brookes: Baltimore

Rubin PN and McCampbell SW (1995) *The Americans with Disabilities Act and Criminal Justice: Mental Disabilities and Corrections*. National Institute of Justice: Washington DC

Rutter M and Plomin R (1997) Opportunities for Psychiatry from Genetic Findings. *British Journal of Psychiatry*, **171**: 209–19

Ryan T (1998) Perceived Risks Associated with Mental Illness: Beyond Homicide and Suicide. *Social Science and Medicine*, **46**(2) 287–97

Sacks O (1985) *The Man Who Mistook His Wife For A Hat*. Picador: London

Sainsbury Centre for Mental Health/Mental Health Act Commission (1997) *Audit of British Acute Psychiatric Hospitals*. Sainsbury Centre for Mental Health: London

SAMHSA (1996) Leaflet: *Before You Label People Look at their Contents*. SAMHSA: Maryland

Sandel M (1981) *Liberalism and the Limits of Justice*. Cambridge University Press: Cambridge

Sandel M (1996) *Democracy's Discontent*. Harvard University Press: Cambridge Massachusetts

Sashidharan S and Francis E (1993) Epidemiology, Ethnicity and Schizophrenia. In Ahmed W (ed.) *Race and Health in Contemporary Britain*. Open University Press: Milton Keynes

Sayce L (1995a) Response to Violence: A Framework for Fair Treatment. In Crichton J (ed.) *Psychiatric Patient Violence*. Duckworth: London

Sayce L (1995b) Campaigning for Change. In Abel A, Buszewicz M, Davison S, Johnson S and Staples E (eds) *Planning Community Mental Health Services for Women*. Routledge: London

Sayce L (1995c) *Breaking the Link Between Homosexuality and Mental Illness. An Unfinished History*. Mind Discussion Document. Mind: London

Sayce L (1996) Good Practice for Women who Have Been Sexually Abused. In Perkins R, Nadirshaw Z, Copperman J and Andrews C (eds) *Women in Context*. Good Practices in Mental Health: London

Sayce L (1997a) Stigma and Social Exclusion: Top Priorities for Policy Makers. *Eurohealth*, Autumn, 5–7

Sayce L (1997b) The War on Drugs and the Efforts to Combat Discrimination Against People Who Take Them. Two Policies at Cross Purposes. Unpublished paper: London

Sayce L (1997c) Motherhood: The Final Taboo in Community Care. *Women and Mental Health Forum*, **2**: 4–7

Sayce L (1998a) Stigma, Discrimination and Social Exclusion: What's in a Word? *Journal of Mental Health, 7*(4): 331–44

Sayce L (1998b) Distress and Disability. *OpenMind*, **89**: 8–9

Sayce L and Measey L (1999) Strategies to Reduce Social Exclusion for People with Mental Health Problems. Editorial, *Psychiatric Bulletin*, **23**(2): 65–7

Sayce L and Willmot J (1997) *Gaining Respect. A Guide to Preventing and Tackling Community Opposition to Mental Health Services*. Mind: London

Sayce L, Craig TKJ and Boardman AP (1991) The Development of Community Mental Health Centres in the UK. *Social Psychiatry and Psychiatric Epidemiology* **26**: 14–20

Schneider EM (1991) The Dialectic of Rights and Politics: Perspectives from the Women's Movement. In Bartlett KT and Kennedy R (eds) *Feminist Legal Theory*. Westview: Boulder, Colorado

Scottish Association for Mental Health (1992) *Community Care and Consultation*. Scottish Association for Mental Health: Edinburgh

Scull A (1995) Paper to Centre for Mental Health Services Annual Congress: Sussex

Secker J (1998) Mental Health Promotion Theory and Practice: Implications for Implementation of Our Healthier Nation. *Mental Health Review*, **3**(2): 5–12

Shakespeare T (1997) Reviewing the Past, Developing the Future. *Skill Journal*, **58**: 8–11

Shapiro JP (1993) *No Pity: People with Disabilities Forging a New Civil Rights Movement*. Times Books: New York

Sharac JS, Yoder B and Sullivan AP (1997) Consumers as Supported Education Mentors. In Mowbray CT, Moxley DP, Jasper CA and Howell LL (eds) *Consumers as Providers of Psychiatric Rehabilitation*. International Association of Psychosocial Rehabilitation Services: Columbia, Maryland

Shaw R (1996) *The Activists' Handbook. A Primer for the 1990s and Beyond*. University of California Press, Berkeley

Shepherd G (1984) *Institutional Care and Rehabilitation*. Longman: London

Sherman PS and Porter R (1991) Mental Health Consumers as Case Management Aides. *Hospital and Community Psychiatry*, **42**: 494–8

Shimrat I (1997) *Call Me Crazy. Stories from the Mad Movement*. Press Gang: Vancouver

Shingler A (1996) Beyond Reason. Exhibition, Mind Annual Conference: Bournemouth

Silverman S (1997) Recovery Through Partnership. On Our Own, Charlottesville, Virginia. In Mowbray CT, Moxley DP, Jasper CA and Howell LL (eds) *Consumers as Providers of Psychiatric Rehabilitation*. International Association of Psychosocial Rehabilitation Services: Columbia, Maryland

Social Exclusion Unit (1998) *Bringing Britain Together: A National Strategy for Neighbourhood Renewal.* Social Exclusion Unit: London

Social Policy Association (1998) Open Letter to Secretary of State for Social Security. *Guardian*, 29 July

Sontag S (1989) *AIDS and its Metaphors.* Allen & Lane: London

Southern Center for Human Rights (1995) Human Rights Report, Fall: Atlanta

Southern Poverty Law Center (1989) *Free At Last. A History of the Civil Rights Movement.* Southern Poverty Law Center: Montgomery, Alabama

Steadman HJ, Robbins PC, Monahan J et al. (1998) *The MacArthur Risk Assessment Study: 1. Executive Summary.* University of Virginia: Charlottesville

Stefan S (1989) Whose Egg Is It Anyway? Reproductive Rights of Incarcerated, Institutionalised and Incompetent Women. *Nova Law Review*, **13**(2): 406–56

Stein L and Test M (1980) Alternatives to Mental Hospital Treatment: Conceptual Model, Treatment Program and Clinical Evaluation. *Archives of General Psychiatry*, **37**: 392–7

Sullivan A (1995) *Virtually Normal: An Argument about Homosexuality.* Alfred A. Knopf: New York

Survivors' Poetry (1996) General Information About Survivors' Poetry: London

Susko MA (ed.) (1991) *Cry of the Invisible. Writings from the Homeless and Survivors of Psychiatric Hospitals.* Conservatory Press: Baltimore

Sutherland P (1987) Backlash. *Disability Rag*, May/June: 1–6

Sweeney M (1997) *Four Perspectives on Mental Illness.* In Mowbray CT, Moxley DP, Jasper CA and Howell LL (eds) *Consumers as Providers of Psychiatric Rehabilitation.* International Association of Psychosocial Rehabilitation Services: Columbia, Maryland

Szasz TS (1971) *The Manufacture of Madness.* Routledge & Kegan Paul: London

Task Force (1990) *From ADA to Empowerment.* Report of the Task Force on the Rights and Empowerment of Americans with Disabilities: Washington DC

Taylor MS and Dear MJ (1981) Scaling Community Attitudes Toward the Mentally Ill. *Schizophrenia Bulletin*, **7**: 225–40

Taylor P and Gunn J (1999) Homicides by People with Mental Illness: Myth and Reality. *British Journal of Psychiatry*, **174**: 9–14

Taylor TL (1992) *Guardians of Hope. The Angels' Guide to Personal Growth.* HJ Kramer: Tiburon, California

Thompson T (1995) *The Beast: A Reckoning with Depression.* Putnam: New York

Tilford S, Delaney F and Vogels M (1997) *Effectiveness of Mental Health Promotion Interventions: A Review.* Health Education Authority: London

Torrey E Fuller, Erdman K, Wolfe SM and Flynn L (1990) *Care of the Seriously Mentally Ill. A Rating of State Programs.* Public Citizen Research Group and National Alliance for the Mentally Ill: Washington DC

Torrey E Fuller, Stieber J, Ezekiel J et al. (1992) Criminalizing the Seriously Mentally Ill: The Abuse of Jails as Mental Hospitals. Public Citizens Health Research Group and the National Alliance for the Mentally Ill: Washington DC

Toscano G and Windau J (1993) Fatal Work Injuries: Results from the 1992 National Census. *Monitor Labor Review*, October, 39–48

Unger K, Anthony WA, Sciarappa MPH and Rogers ES (1991) A Supported Education Program for Young Adults with Long-term Mental Illness. *Hospital and Community Psychiatry*, **42**(8): 838–42

United Nations (1992) The Protection of Persons with Mental Illness and the Improvement of Mental Health Care. Resolution Adopted by the General Assembly 46/119. United Nations: New York

United Nations (1993) Standard Rules on the Equalisation of Opportunity for Disabled People. United Nations: New York

United Nations (1994) General Comment on People with Disabilities. United Nations: New York

United States Holocaust Memorial Museum (1996) *Handicapped*. United States Holocaust Memorial Museum: Washington DC

Unzicker R (1994) On My Own. A Personal Journey Through Madness and Re-emergence. In Spaniol L and Koehler M (eds) *The Experience of Recovery*. Center for Psychiatric Rehabilitation: Boston

Vaccaro V (1991) Reasonable Accommodations for People with Mental Disabilities. *Policy in Perspective*, November/December: 10–11

Vaid U (1995) *Virtual Equality: The Mainstreaming of Gay and Lesbian Liberation*. Anchor Doubleday: New York

Vedder R (1996) The Split Level Society. *Washington Post*, 16 June: 10

Vernon A (1995) Understanding Simultaneous Oppression. Disability Rights, A Symposium of the European Regions. European Day of Disabled Persons: Southampton

Wahl OF (1993) Community Impact of Group Homes for Mentally Ill Adults. *Community Mental Health Journal*, **29**(3): 247–59

Wahl OF (1995) *Media Madness. Public Images of Mental Illness*. Rutgers University Press: New Jersey

Wallcraft J (1996) Becoming Fully Ourselves. In Read J and Reynolds J (eds) *Speaking Our Minds*. Open University Press/Macmillan: Basingstoke

Wallcraft J (1999) Healing Minds. A Report on Current Research, Policy and Practice Concerning the Use of Complementary and Alternative Therapies for a Wide Range of Mental Health Problems. Mental Health Foundation: London

Warner R (1985) *Recovery from Schizophrenia. Psychiatry and Political Economy*. Routledge: London

Warner R (1996) The Cultural Context of Mental Distress. In Heller T, Reynolds J, Gomm R, Muston R and Pattison S (eds) *Mental Health Matters. A Reader*. Open University/Macmillan: Basingstoke

Watson D (1993) A Study in Legislative Strategy. The Passage of the ADA. In Gostin LO and Beyer JD (eds) *Implementing the Americans with Disabilities Act. Rights and Responsibilities of All Americans*. Brookes, Baltimore

Webb-Johnson A (1991) *A Cry for Change. An Asian Perspective on Developing Quality Mental Health Care*. Confederation of Indian Organisations: London

Wellcome Trust (1997) Cracked. Teachers' Pack. Science Through the Arts. Wellcome Trust: London

West C (1994) *Race Matters*. Vintage Books: New York

West C and Gates HL (1996) *The Future of the Race*. Alfred A Knopf: New York

West J (1996) *Implementing the Americans with Disabilities Act*. Blackwell: Cambridge, Massachusetts

Wheatcroft G (1998) Annus Memorabilis. *Prospect*, January: 25–8

Whittle L (1998) One Woman's Experience of the Survivor Movement. *Women and Mental Health Forum*, **3**: 12

Wilden A (1972) *System and Structure. Essays in Communication and Exchange*. Tavistock: London

Wilkinson RG (1996) *Unhealthy Societies. The Afflictions of Inequality.* Routledge: London

Williams PJ (1995) *The Rooster's Egg. On the Persistence of Prejudice.* Harvard University Press: Cambridge, Massachusetts

Williams X (1995) Some Disabilities Are More Equal Than Others. *Disability Rag and ReSource,* March/April: 6–9

Wilson M (1997) Printing it in Black and White. *OpenMind,* **85**: 16–17

Wilson M and Francis J (1997) *Raised Voices.* Mind: London

Wing JK and Morris B (1981) *Handbook of Psychiatric Rehabilitation.* Oxford University Press: Oxford

Wolff G, Pathare S, Craig T and Leff J (1996a) Public Education for Community Care. *British Journal of Psychiatry,* **168**: 441–7

Wolff G, Pathare S, Craig T and Leff J (1996b) Community Attitudes to Mental Illness. *British Journal of Psychiatry,* **168**: 183–90

Women Against Rape/Legal Action for Women (1995) Dossier: *The Crown Prosecution Service and the Crime of Rape.* Women Against Rape: London

World Mental Health Day (1997) Information Pack. Children and Mental Health. World Federation for Mental Health. Co-sponsored by World Health Organisation: Virginia

Yates K (1995) Moving out of Isolation. In Grobe J (ed.) *Beyond Bedlam, Contemporary Women Psychiatric Survivors Speak Out.* Third Side Press: Chicago

Yuker HE (1988) Perceptions of Severely and Multiply Disabled Persons. *Journal of the Multihandicapped Person,* **1**(1): 5–16

Zeitz MA (1995) The Mothers' Project: a Clinical Case Management System. *Psychiatric Rehabilitation Journal,* **19**(1): 55–62

Zinman S, Howie the Harp and Budd S (1987) *Reaching Across. Mental Health Clients Helping Each Other.* California Network of Mental Health Clients: Sacramento

Zito Trust (1997) *Zito Monitor 2.* Zito Trust: London

Index